THE UNIVERSITY OF LIVERPOOL

HAROLD COHEN LIBRARY

Removable Partial Dentures

Quintessentials of Dental Practice – 18
Prosthodontics - 3

Removable Partial Dentures

By
Nicholas J A Jepson

Editor-in-Chief: Nairn H F Wilson
Editor Prosthodontics: P Finbarr Allen

Quintessence Publishing Co. Ltd.
London, Berlin, Chicago, Copenhagen, Paris, Milan, Barcelona,
Istanbul, São Paulo, Tokyo, New Delhi, Moscow, Prague, Warsaw

British Library Cataloguing in Publication Data

Jepson, N. J. A.
    Removable partial dentures. – (Quintessentials of dental practice;
    18. Prosthodontics; 3)
    1. Partial dentures, removable
    I. Title II. Wilson, Nairn H. F. III. Allen, P. Finbarr
    617.6´92

    ISBN 1850970750

Copyright © 2004 Quintessence Publishing Co. Ltd., London

ISBN 1-85097-075-0

Dedicated to my family and my patients.

Foreword

Success in partial denture prosthodontics – in addition to being a real practice-builder – can be very satisfying. The art and science of partial denture prosthodontics may, however, be viewed as complex and challenging. But, as with most things in dentistry, and as is emphasised in this most welcome addition to the *Quintessentials of Dental Practice Series*, success in the provision of partial dentures is dependent on the adherence to a number of inescapable, underpinning principles: good diagnosis, including an understanding of the patient's needs and expectations, knowledge and understanding of the capabilities of existing materials and techniques, careful planning and attention to detail. Equally important is the need to control and treat active oral disease prior to embarking on the replacement of missing teeth – a principle which the author of this carefully crafted, succinct text rightfully places great importance on.

Turning to practical matters, this book provides the practitioner with evidence-based guidelines directly applicable to everyday clinical practice. Of particular note is the sound, easy-to-follow and refreshingly pragmatic approach to partial denture design – an element of partial denture provision which must be undertaken by the practitioner if the completed dentures are to be acceptable and pleasing to the patient, let alone perform well in clinical service. If you suspect that many of your partial dentures – in particular, your lower free-end saddle – dentures spend most of their time in a jar, or worse have been lost at the back of some bathroom cabinet or other domestic black hole for items which appeared to be a good idea, but proved to be of little, if any, practical value, then you should read this book. If partial dentures are worth making, then they are worth making well – the thrust of this insightful book.

As you would expect of a volume in the *Quintessentials of Dental Practice Series*, this book is extensively illustrated with high-quality images and produced to an excellent standard. Few, if any, other books on partial dentures provides so much information in a text which may take only an evening or two to read and digest. Your partially dentate patients would be very pleased to hear that this book has formed part of your Continuing Professional Development.

Nairn Wilson
Editor-in-Chief

Preface

A partial denture may be defined as a removable prosthesis that replaces a missing tooth or teeth and associated supporting tissues in an arch where some natural teeth remain. It is one of the means of restoring the dental appearance and function for patients with missing teeth and, where such a need exists, there is strong evidence to support their successful use in the long-term.

In terms of materials and techniques very little has changed in recent years in the clinical provision of partial dentures. What has changed significantly is the context of this provision and our understanding of its effects. Important and continuing demographic changes of the partially dentate population, the increasing availability of alternative treatments and, above all, a substantial and growing evidence base for the long-term effectiveness of partial dentures are now significant influences on their use. This book presents a review of these influences and, based on evidence, a systematic and effective approach to removable partial denture provision.

Having Read This Book

It is hoped that after reading this book the reader will:
- Recognise the demographic changes to the partially dentate population, and appreciate the effectiveness of partial dentures and the consequences of their use.
- Understand the clinical and patient-related factors that indicate the use of partial dentures and recognise the need to base the provision of partial dentures on perceived aesthetic and functional needs of the patient.
- Recognise that not all missing teeth need to be replaced and be aware of the concept of functionally oriented treatment planning for the partially dentate.
- Understand the basic principles of partial denture design and the application of these principles to the design of the several partial denture components.
- Understand the procedure of cast surveying and how this may be applied to the process of a simple and practical system of design for effective partial dentures.

- Recognise that the design of partial dentures is the responsibility of the dental practitioner.
- Be aware of the clinical techniques and materials used in the construction of partial dentures.
- Understand the indications for and types of transitional partial dentures.

Nicholas J A Jepson

Acknowledgements

My thanks are due to Mr Dean Barker, Professor Bengt Öwall, Mr David Smith, and Mr Richard Tones for permission to use some of their photographs as illustrations in the text. I must also acknowledge the role played by my many past and present colleagues, patients and students in forming my views on treatment of the partially dentate in general and the use of partial dentures in particular.

Contents

Chapter 1
Partial Denture Provision

Aim

In industrialised countries, as the proportion of adults retaining some of their teeth into old age increases, so will the likely need for prosthetic intervention. This chapter aims to provide an overview of the need and demand for partial dentures to restore partially dentate adults.

Outcome

After reading this chapter the practitioner should be aware of the effectiveness and consequences of partial denture use.

The Partially Dentate Population

Evidence from various national dental health surveys in developed countries clearly indicates that the proportion of people with no teeth at all will continue to decline and that more people will retain some of their own teeth into old age. The results of the 1998 national dental health survey in the UK indicate that 87% of all adults had some natural teeth but that this proportion was strongly influenced by age. The mean number of missing teeth by age group for a number of developed countries is shown in Fig 1-1 using data from the WHO Collaborating Centre, Sweden (2003). Common trends are that significant tooth loss only becomes apparent after 45 years of age and that the number of missing teeth increases with age. The percentage of people ≥ 45 years of age provided with partial dentures differs between countries, a variation that reflects both differing public and professional attitudes to partial denture use and healthcare systems, but can reach levels of 20–30%. Where provision of partial dentures is a commonly used treatment option for the partially dentate, the principal deciding factor as to whether or not a partial denture is used appears to be the number of remaining natural teeth. Results of the 1998 UK Dental Health Survey clearly indicate that there is a cut-off point at 21–24 teeth and people with 21 or more teeth are unlikely to have removable partial dentures (Fig 1-2). This supports the important concept of a "functional dentition" which allows the patient sufficient function and comfort without the need for tooth replacements.

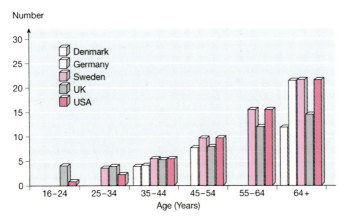

Fig 1-1 The mean number of missing teeth by age group (data from WHO Collaborating Centre, Malmö, Sweden 2003).

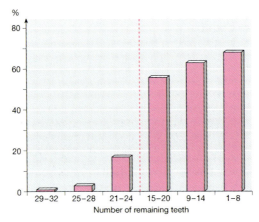

Fig 1-2 The proportion of partially dentate adults with removable partial dentures by number of natural teeth (Adult Dental Health Survey, Oral Health in the United Kingdom 1998).

The number of teeth that people retain has also increased. In the UK in 1998, over 72% of adults had 21 or more teeth although this figure reduced with age such that only 10% of people aged ≥75 years had 21 or more teeth. Projections for 2018 suggest that 90% of 16–74 year olds in the UK will have a natural dentition of 21 or more teeth though this proportion will again reduce with age. Such projections need to be seen in the context of increasing life span in industrialised countries with an increasing percentage of populations ≥65 years old. In the UK, for example, the number of adults over the age of 65 years is expected to rise by 2.7 million by 2021.

Increased tooth retention reflects the development of more positive attitudes to dental health and improved access to dental care. Adults increasingly wish to retain their natural teeth and are prepared to accept treatment recommended by their dentists to save their teeth. There is good evidence that dental attendance improves the possibility of retaining at least some teeth over the course of a lifetime. Increasingly, adults find the prospect of complete dentures unacceptable though, interestingly, such attitudes do not seem to apply to the use of partial dentures. The future then is one of increasing numbers of older partially dentate adults who may require partial dentures to replace missing teeth.

Projections based on data from national surveys have been used to estimate the future treatment need for the partially dentate. These estimates point to an increased need for both fixed and removable prosthesis. In the USA the projected total need for fixed and removable prosthesis is put at 115% of current provision by the year 2020. Partial dentures are the simplest, cheapest and by far the most common method of replacing missing teeth. In the UK approximately 30% of all middle aged and elderly adults have been provided with partial dentures. There is, however, an increasing acceptance of the use of fixed prosthesis by elderly patients and a growing recognition that implant-supported prosthesis offer a viable and, perhaps, more effective long-term treatment alternative for the partially dentate. Socio-economic factors would suggest, however, that the more frequent use of partial dentures will remain the situation for the foreseeable future. This together with the evident population trends would suggest that the need for partial dentures in developed countries is unlikely to decrease in the future and will probably remain relatively stable.

The Effectiveness of Partial Denture Provision

For the very large majority of cases, partial dentures are provided to improve appearance by restoring visible spaces resulting from the loss of typically anterior teeth and to improve function by restoring missing posterior, usually molar, teeth. In addition, the use of partial dentures is often advocated to maintain occlusal stability. This section will review the effectiveness of partial denture use in these circumstances.

Appearance

The improved appearance gained by the replacement of missing anterior teeth really needs no amplification (Fig 1-3). It is probably the main reason patients request partial dentures and, perhaps, continue to wear them but this is not inevitably the case. There is good evidence to suggest that the dentist's

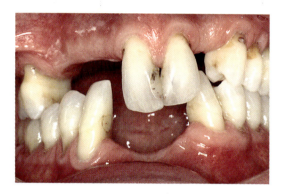

Fig 1-3 The presence of visible spaces because of missing anterior teeth is likely to be the main factor motivating this patient to seek treatment to replace them.

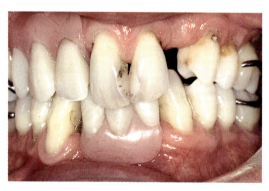

Fig 1-4 Somewhat surprisingly, the patient was insistent that the missing UL2 should not be replaced.

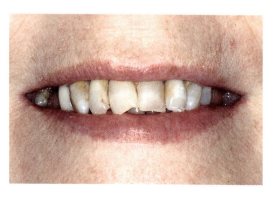

Fig 1-5 Many elderly patients find the presence of visible spaces quite acceptable.

and patient's view of what is or is not a satisfactory appearance can differ markedly (Fig 1-4). The key factor is, of course, the patient's opinion and this is strongly linked to what they perceive is an acceptable appearance in their social environment, a concept of social ease and acceptability well described by social scientists as "passing". The age of the patient does seem to influence the importance attached to appearance. For younger patients, the loss of visible teeth is likely to be unacceptable and a powerful driving force to seek treatment, yet many elderly patients can find the presence of visible spaces resulting, for example, from the loss of first premolar teeth quite acceptable (Fig 1-5). As age increases there appears to be a greater focus on the need for acceptable function rather than appearance.

Masticatory function

The classic description of the possible effects of a reducing number of natural teeth on masticatory function is shown in Fig 1-6. Tooth loss, in particular that of posterior teeth, results in difficulty chewing and biting food – that is a limitation of masticatory function. This in turn leads to changes in food choices, an impaired dietary intake that may be associated with nutritional deficiency. Replacement of missing teeth restores masticatory function and allows the patient more dietary freedom and the possibility to improve dietary intake.

It was for many years a basic assumption that the progressive loss of posterior teeth would reduce chewing efficiency to the extent that problems of digestion would ensue. Indeed, there is evidence to suggest that as teeth are lost so objective measures of masticatory performance deteriorate. However, many patients with large numbers of missing posterior teeth have little or no complaint about their ability to chew food. They have no perceived functional limitation and, indeed, the poor correlation between objective and

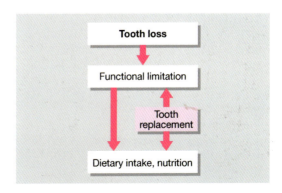

Fig 1-6 The possible effects of a reducing number of natural teeth on masticatory function.

5

subjective assessments of masticatory function is a common research finding. Recent research suggests that patients can masticate adequately without molars and even second premolars, the assumption being that they compensate for a poor occlusion by swallowing larger particles of food rather than chewing for longer. The factor determining whether a patient perceives a limitation of masticatory function appears to be the number of pairs of occluding posterior teeth. Evidence suggests that unless the patient has fewer than three occluding pairs of posterior teeth there is no socio-functional benefit to be gained from replacing missing molar teeth in shortened dental arches. Assuming no loss of anterior teeth, this equates to a "functional threshold" of 21 or more teeth with three to five pairs of occluding posterior teeth – the "functional dentition" referred to earlier in the chapter.

The relationship between limitation of masticatory function resulting from tooth loss and impaired dietary intake has been established but much less clearly for the partially dentate than it has been for the edentulous. The indications are that the number and distribution of teeth are strongly associated with dietary intake. For example, the probability of achieving the recommended daily intake of a number of fruit and vegetables and that the measured intake of dietary fibre and vitamin C appears to fall with reducing numbers of pairs of occluding posterior teeth.

Although an improved masticatory function following the replacement of missing posterior teeth should allow more dietary freedom, there is no evidence that an improved dietary intake will be achieved unless treatment is accompanied by dietary advice. Clearly dietary habits do not simply reflect masticatory function. Other lifestyle and socio-economic factors are important influences and may, indeed, be associated with the loss of teeth in the first place. Given that the evidence for the effects of tooth loss on masticatory function and dietary intake is drawn almost exclusively from the developed countries, such findings are perhaps unsurprising. The less challenging nature of diets in industrialised societies means that nutrition and survival are no longer questions of masticatory function.

Maintaining occlusal stability
Loss of teeth can result in the loss of stable occlusal contacts between opposing teeth and contacts between adjacent teeth. This may lead to undesirable movements such as tilting, drifting and over eruption of teeth (Fig 1-7). Patients may seek a new occlusal position to maximise tooth contacts. This may then lead to abnormal loading of teeth and their further movement – a loss of occlusal stability. Replacement of missing teeth will prevent these unwanted move-

ments and maintain occlusal stability in the long-term. However, patients will often seek treatment some years after the loss of teeth. Some movement of teeth may have already occurred and a new intercuspal relationship, often less desirable but nonetheless stable, established. The horse has bolted and shutting the stable door by replacing the missing teeth cannot be justified. Further these movements of teeth are not inevitable. They are seen more frequently in the young and, when seen in the adult, are more commonly associated with periodontally involved teeth. Where oral hygiene is adequate, it is the clinical experience of many practitioners that the position of teeth will remain quite stable.

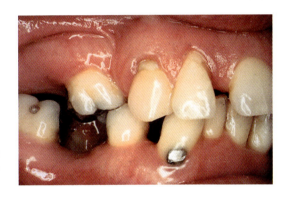

Fig 1-7 Tooth movements following the loss of stable occlusal contacts.

Loss of posterior teeth results in an increased use of anterior teeth during mastication with, it is said, possible overloading of the temporomandibular apparatus. In addition, altered patterns of muscular function may result from the movement of teeth as the patient attempts to avoid abnormal contacts and seeks a new position of maximum intercuspation. The consequence is said to be an increased predisposition to temporomandibular joint dysfunction. Whilst the correction of abnormal occlusal contacts and replacement of missing teeth still feature in the treatment of patients with symptoms of temporomandibular dysfunction, evidence supporting an association between the loss of posterior teeth and the development of symptoms of temporomandibular dysfunction is lacking.

Consequences of Partial Denture Use

The possible consequences of the provision of partial dentures can be considered under the following headings:
• patient acceptance
• long-term effects.

Patient acceptance

Although their widespread use continues at considerable cost, past studies have established rates of patient non-use of partial dentures that range from 10 to 60%, irrespective of any intended benefit to appearance and function. The wide variation in reported acceptance rates probably reflects differing study numbers, patient types and assessment methods but a feature emphasised in many of these reports is the absence of common clinical factors to explain non-acceptance. What is clear is that there is a significant divergence between clinical intent and treatment outcome as measured by the prevalence of partial denture use. Together with the potential of partial dentures to generate an additional long-term treatment need, this represents, at best, a considerable potential waste of resource. For a significant number of patients the perception of the need for or benefit of partial dentures differs from that of the clinician.

It is tempting to ascribe non-use of partial dentures solely to deficiencies in their design. Clearly, patients find difficulty tolerating dentures that are ill-fitting, broken or interfere with normal occlusal contacts. However, assuming the adequacy of their construction, there is no strong evidence that aspects of design, e.g., material, Kennedy classification and connector type, are important influences on patient acceptance. The only clearly established predictor for partial denture use is the presence of anterior replacement teeth. Denture materials (acrylic or metal), design and location did influence attitudes to partial denture use but to a much smaller extent. It does appear that the main driver for acceptance and use of partial dentures is a perceived functional gain by the patient. If no functional benefit is perceived, then the patient decides that the inconvenience is not worth it and stops wearing them.

Long-term effects

The possible advantage of improved appearance and function offered by partial dentures should be balanced against their long-term potential to cause harm to the remaining teeth and supporting soft tissues. In broad terms this harm can be described as a risk of local damage to the remaining teeth resulting from an increased incidence of caries and periodontal disease and the continued resorption of those parts of the alveolar process supporting the partial denture.

Caries and periodontal disease

The subjective clinical findings pointing to an association between the use of partial dentures and deteriorating caries and periodontal status of the

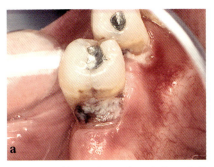 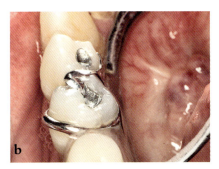

Fig 1-8 (a,b) Caries and periodontal disease apparently associated with the use of a partial denture.

remaining natural teeth have been of longstanding concern (Fig 1-8). Well-conducted controlled clinical trials and findings from large epidemiological surveys have established this association and there is now a powerful evidence base for an increased incidence of caries and, to a lesser extent, periodontal disease in patients wearing partial dentures. These findings can be summarised as follows:

- Abutment teeth were more likely to have caries and periodontal disease than all other teeth.
- In the elderly, the presence of a partial denture was strongly associated with root surface caries. This finding is of particular concern given that the partially dentate tend to be elderly and that the management of root caries is at best difficult if not intractable.
- The relative risk of new caries was approximately four times greater for patients wearing partial dentures than in those with fixed prosthesis.
- Root caries and periodontal diseases were more frequent when the partial denture was defective.
- The increased incidence of caries in partial denture wearers was independent of patient demographic factors and other caries risk factors such as sugar intake and salivary flow.
- High levels of plaque control can offset the increased incidence of caries and periodontal disease – that is, a partial denture *per se* will not cause carious and periodontal lesions.

Plaque and partial dentures
Dental plaque is the main aetiologic factor in both caries and periodontal disease. Given that the use of partial dentures in the absence of effective plaque control increases the incidence of caries and periodontal disease, the sugges-

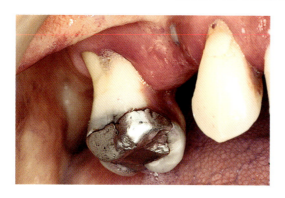

Fig 1-9 Plaque formation on surfaces adjacent to a partial denture.

tion is that this change occurs through an effect of partial dentures on plaque formation. The relationship between partial dentures and plaque has been the subject of numerous investigations and their findings are as follows:

- Partial dentures do adversely affect plaque formation by increasing its amount and altering the pattern of its deposition and probably the type of plaque formed. The increase in plaque formation was greater on tooth surfaces adjacent to and covered by the partial denture and was also apparent on teeth free from the partial denture (Fig 1-9).
- Normal toothbrushing did not offset the increase in plaque seen when partial dentures were worn. The implication is that a level of plaque control deemed "adequate" without a partial denture may not remain so when a partial denture is worn. In particular, proximal surfaces adjacent to denture bases and other surfaces covered by denture components should be pointed out to patients as surfaces to which they must give special attention. Additional cleaning aids will normally be required and patients should be advised about them and their use demonstrated.

Changes to the alveolar process
Resorption of the supporting alveolar process is a frequent clinical finding. Common consequences are reduced retention, instability, loss of occlusal contacts and fracture of denture components. Further, trauma from the resulting ill-fitting dentures may well cause inflammation of the denture-bearing mucosa. Such trauma and an overgrowth of the fungus *Candida albicans* are thought to be the most common causes of denture-induced stomatitis not infrequently seen under ill-fitting upper dentures.

The question as to whether there is a cause–effect relationship between this resorptive process and denture use has not been clearly answered. Although several studies strongly suggest this relationship, the small study populations and the large individual variations seen have cast doubt on the validity of the results. There is no evidence for the concept of disuse atrophy in non-denture wearers.

Key Points

- More people will retain some of their own teeth into old age and the number of teeth retained will increase.
- The future need for partial dentures to restore aesthetic and functional limitations will increase.
- The long-term use of partial dentures is associated with an increased incidence of caries and periodontal disease.
- Replacement of missing front teeth is the main factor motivating the use of partial dentures. Improved mastication is of secondary importance.
- The provision of partial dentures should be based on a patient's perceived need.

References

Kelly M, Steele JG, Nuttall N, et al. Adult Dental Health Survey UK 1998. London: Office for National Statistics, 2000.

WHO Oral Health Country Profile. Sweden: WHO Collaborating Centre, Malmö University, 2003.

Further Reading

Jepson NJ, Moynihan PJ, Kelly PJ, et al. Caries incidence following restoration of shortened lower dental arches in a randomised controlled trial. Br Dent J 2001;191:140–144.

Sheiham A, Steele JG, Marcenes W, et al. The relationship among dental status, nutrient intake, and nutritional status in older people. J Dent Res 2001;80:408–413.

Steele JG, Treasure E, Pitts NB, et al. Total tooth loss in the United Kingdom in 1998 and implications for the future. Br Dent J 2000;189:598–603.

Chapter 2
Indications for Partial Dentures

Aim

This chapter aims to describe the clinical and patient-related factors that indicate the use of partial dentures to restore partially dentate patients. In addition, it will emphasise the need to base the provision of partial dentures on perceived aesthetic and functional needs and introduce the practitioner to the concept of functionally oriented treatment planning for the partially dentate.

Outcome

After reading this chapter, the practitioner should be aware that missing teeth do not always need to be replaced and that the effective provision of partial dentures should be based on the establishment of patient need. Once this need has been established, there are clear clinical and patient-related factors that indicate the use of partial dentures in preference to other treatment options including fixed prosthesis and implant-supported prosthesis.

Treatment Options

When formulating treatment plans for partially dentate patients, several treatment options may be possible for the replacement of missing teeth (Box 2-1). A number of clinical and patient-related factors will suggest the use of partial dentures, and these will be described in later sections of this chapter. However, it should be emphasised that the first question to be considered is whether or not any missing teeth should be replaced.

Reasons Not to Provide Partial Dentures

Traditionally, the replacement of all missing teeth was thought necessary to preserve function and maintain occlusal stability – the concept of arch integrity. Whilst it is invariably possible to replace missing teeth, the evidence clearly indicates that replacement must be based on self-perceived aesthetic and functional needs by the patient – a functionally oriented approach. The evidence described in Chapter 1 clearly indicates that the failure to base

Box 2-1

Treatment Options for the Replacement of Missing Teeth
No replacement
Fixed prosthesis (conventional, adhesive or hybrid)
Partial dentures
Implant-supported prosthesis (fixed or removable)
A combination of fixed and removable prosthesis

partial denture provision on a perceived need will, at best, result in the denture not being worn and, at worst, result in an additional treatment need through harm to and the possible future loss of remaining teeth. This evidence, together with the predictions for increasing numbers of older partially dentate adults, indicates that new treatment strategies are required to meet the demands of the future elderly population. This is particularly so when there are increasing pressures to ensure the effective use of health resources which are not only finite but may also decrease with time.

A functionally oriented approach

Current research suggests that the replacement of all missing teeth is unnecessary and at times inadvisable. Many patients and, in particular elderly patients, can function adequately, if suboptimally, without the replacement of missing posterior teeth. Evidence describes such a "functional dentition" as one with 21 or more teeth or, more specifically, one with at least three pairs of opposing posterior teeth.

A functionally oriented approach is one in which teeth are replaced only in response to an established patient need. The shortened dental arch (SDA) concept is one example of this approach, which is, in particular, applicable to the elderly and where limited finance is available for restorative care. Treatment effort and resources are directed at solving patients' problems and are targeted on preserving those teeth necessary to meet the patients' aesthetic and functional needs. This normally implies that treatment is focused on maintaining anterior and premolar teeth (Fig 2-1). Molars are replaced only if their absence causes problems to the patient and thus the use of partial dentures is avoided if possible. Appropriate case selection is essential for the successful application of the SDA approach. The main requirements for the

SDA approach are (i) the long-term prognosis for the remaining anterior and premolar teeth should be good and (ii) the patient is motivated to maintain them. Although the future loss of one or two of the remaining teeth can be accommodated by the use of simple fixed prosthesis, the continued loss of teeth will compromise appearance and function. Contraindications to the SDA approach are given in Box 2-2.

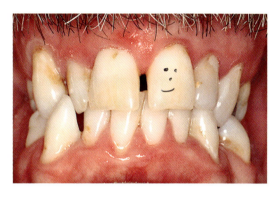

Fig 2-1 A shortened dental arch. Future treatment will be directed at maintaining the function of the remaining anterior and premolar teeth.

Box 2-2

Shortened Dental Arch Approach: Contraindications

Severe Class II or Class III incisal relationships
Pre-existing temporomandibular dysfunction
Advanced pathological wear
Advanced periodontal disease
Patient is under the age of 40 years
Parafunction

A functionally orientated approach will result in a reduced but more effective provision of partial dentures. It may also indicate that treatment options other than the use of partial dentures to replace missing teeth are more appropriate. An example of this approach is shown in Fig 2-2.

When to Use Partial Dentures

Having established the need to replace missing teeth, from a mechanistic and functional viewpoint, it could be argued that a fixed or implant-supported

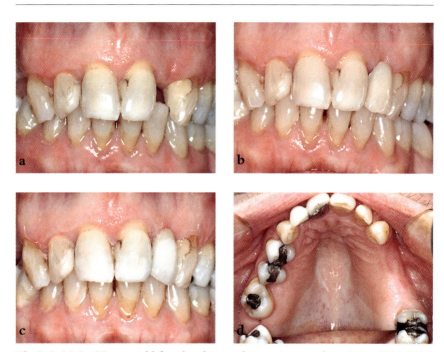

Fig 2-2 (a) An 80-year-old female whose only concern was the missing UL2. UL2 and other missing upper teeth are replaced by an upper partial denture (b). The patient had no complaint about the fit of the denture but restricted its use to social occasions and avoided using it for eating because it interfered with taste and felt bulky. The remaining teeth were sound. (c,d) The upper partial denture was replaced by a simple cantilever resin-bonded bridge restoring the missing UL2.

prosthesis will always be the treatment of choice and that a partial denture is indicated only when alternative treatments are contraindicated. In some respects this is true, in particular with regard to fixed prostheses where their use may be considered to be limited by the suitability of potential abutment teeth and the length of the edentulous span. Where the use of either a fixed or removable prosthesis is equally feasible, other patient-related factors may suggest the use of partial dentures. The indications for the use of partial dentures are considered separately in the following sections. In reality they are not mutually exclusive and there is considerable overlap.

Number and distribution of missing teeth
Factors of particular importance are the length and number of edentulous spaces. Partial dentures are strongly indicated when the loss of teeth is

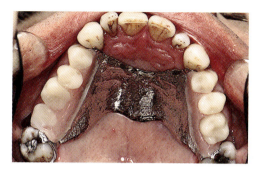

Fig 2-3 Use of an upper partial denture to replace effectively two bounded posterior saddles.

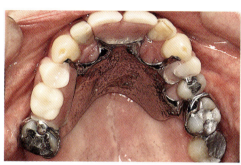

Fig 2-4 Use of a partial denture to restore combined anterior and posterior tooth loss.

restricted to long edentulous bounded saddles. In posterior segments, this usually means contiguous spans of at least three teeth and reflects the increasing difficulties of identifying suitable abutments for fixed prosthesis for spans of this length. Where two such contiguous spans are located bilaterally, partial dentures can offer a simple and effective means of tooth replacement that demonstrates their particular advantage of joining a number of edentulous spaces into one functional unit (Fig 2-3). Single anterior edentulous spaces up to and including the four incisor teeth are most effectively restored using fixed prostheses. Use of partial dentures in such circumstances can result in a compromised appearance and difficulty ensuring denture stability, in particular when patients incise food. As the length of the anterior saddle increases to include replacement of canine and then premolar teeth, so does the indication for the use of partial dentures. Partial dentures are indicated when extensive anterior and posterior tooth loss occurs in combination and their particular attribute simultaneously to restore different edentulous spaces is again demonstrated (Fig 2-4).

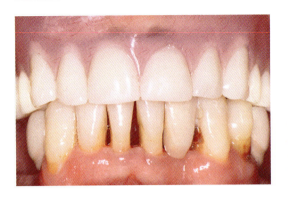

Fig 2-5 Resin-bonded bridgework replacing LL5, LL2 and LR4 to restore a shortened lower dental arch opposing a complete upper denture.

Severely shortened dental arches are frequently associated with complaints of difficulties in biting and chewing food and have traditionally been restored using free-end saddle partial dentures. Where a severely shortened lower dental arch opposes a complete upper denture, a lower free-end saddle denture provides occlusal stability through the distribution of contacts around the arch. This is said to contribute to the continued stability and retention of the complete upper denture and avoids the potential for rapid and continued resorption of the anterior upper edentulous ridge often described as the "combination syndrome". More recent evidence suggests that, in the elderly, restoration with single-pontic distal cantilever fixed prosthesis of conventional or adhesive design can be a more effective solution even when the lower SDA is opposed by a complete denture. This is only possible if there are sufficient remaining suitable abutment teeth to allow restoration of a contiguous SDA of at least eight teeth (Fig 2-5). If this is not the case, restoration should be effected with a partial denture although the use of implant-supported prosthesis may also be considered.

Partial dentures are unsuited to the restoration of one or two-tooth anterior or posterior spaces where their bulk, potential for movement and relative complexity of design can offset any aesthetic or functional gain. In such circumstances, fixed prostheses are the treatment of choice. Partial dentures should, however, be considered where several short spans are to be restored. In such circumstances, partial dentures offer a simple alternative to potentially complex fixed restorations (Fig 2-6).

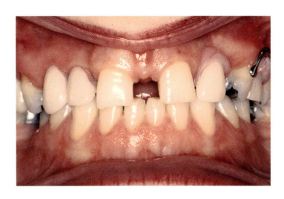

Fig 2-6 An upper partial denture replacing several short edentulous spans.

Status of potential abutment teeth

Relevant factors include the alignment, restorative status and prognosis of potential abutment teeth. The unfavourable alignment of potential abutments can preclude the use of a fixed prosthesis through the need to remove extensive amounts of tooth tissue to establish a usable path of insertion (Fig 2-7). There is an increasing reluctance to prepare previously unrestored teeth for a conventional fixed prosthesis, in particular, in younger patients. The loss of sound tooth tissue is irreversible and, although evidence suggests that the survival rates for a clinically excellent fixed prosthesis can be ≥15 years, failure is often catastrophic and can result in the loss of abutment teeth. Adhesive fixed prosthesis may offer a solution for the restoration of short edentulous spans up to a maximum of two teeth (Fig 2-8). Abutment teeth of poor prognosis put the long-term success of fixed prostheses at risk – in particular those that are extensive and complex. Other risk factors include previous or required extensive restoration, the adequacy of or need for endodontic treatment and a poor or unstable periodontal status. In such circumstances, partial dentures can offer a simpler, pragmatic and effective means of replacing teeth.

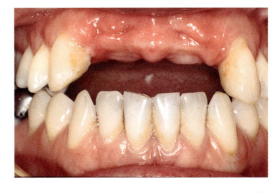

Fig 2-7 Alignment of the upper canines precludes the use of a conventional fixed bridge.

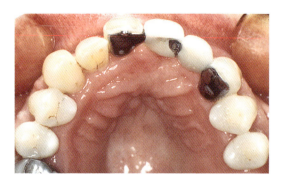

Fig 2-8 Use of two cantilever resin-bonded bridges to restore a two-tooth edentulous span.

Soft tissue loss

The traumatic loss of teeth or the continued resorption of the edentulous ridge may be associated with significant loss of the supporting soft tissues (Fig 2-9a). Failure to restore the vertical and horizontal deficiencies in the soft tissue contour resulting from tissue loss in the anterior segment will result in a poor appearance due to incorrect tooth position and inadequate lip support. Fixed prosthesis cannot adequately restore extensive soft tissue loss which is best effected with partial dentures where the saddle acrylic and flange can be easily modified to replace lost soft tissue, allow the correct positioning of replacement teeth and restore labial fullness (Fig 2-9b).

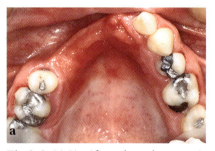
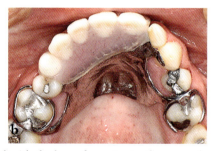

Fig 2-9 (a) Significant bone loss associated with the loss of anterior teeth as a result of trauma. (b) Restoration of the lost tissue with a partial denture saddle allows the correct positioning of replacement anterior teeth and normal labial support.

Anterior tooth spacing

Restoration of an acceptable appearance may require the use of spaced anterior teeth (Fig 2-10). The reproduction of a midline diastema between two or more replacement incisor teeth will normally preclude the use of a fixed prosthesis and appearance is simply and effectively restored with a partial denture. In the particular circumstance of the replacement of a single anterior tooth with spacing, fixed and removable options are possible but far from ideal and the most effective treatment option is the single-tooth implant (Fig 2-11).

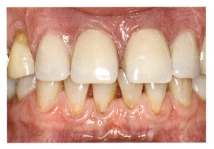

Fig 2-10 An acceptable arrangement of the replacement anterior teeth required inclusion of a midline diastema.

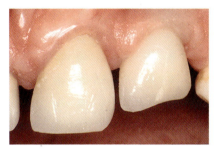

Fig 2-11 A single-tooth implant replacing the missing UL2 with spacing. (Courtesy of Mr DG Smith.)

Restoration of occlusal face height

The loss of posterior tooth contacts as a consequence of damaging periodontal or occlusal factors can result in the loss of occlusal face height with anterior teeth becoming proclined and splayed (bite collapse) or heavily worn (Fig 2-12). If anterior contact is absent overclosure with trauma to the palatal tissues will result. The ideal treatment for such patients is often to restore and stabilise the occlusal face height with partial dentures that replace the missing posterior teeth and overlay worn teeth if necessary (Fig 2-13). Such dentures may be used as the definitive restoration or as an interim prosthesis that acts to restore appearance and provide occlusal stability before the provision of definitive fixed or removable prosthesis.

Patient preference and cost

The final arbiter in the choice of treatment is clearly the patient. Prior to making treatment decisions the patient must be fully informed of the procedures and costs involved in the various treatment options and their likely effectiveness and outcome. Although the choices of treatment will reflect individual preference, some general trends are there. Evidence indicates that younger patients prefer to avoid the use of partial dentures. For the elderly, frailty, poor general health and non-independent living may preclude more

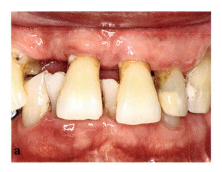

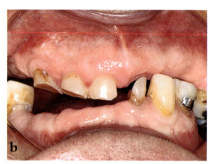

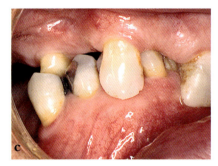

Fig 2-12 Loss of occlusal face height associated with various combinations of loss of tooth contacts, wear and periodontal disease. (a) Splaying of the remaining anterior teeth is evident as is (b,c) the potential for palatal soft tissue trauma.

time consuming and demanding clinical procedures associated with the use of fixed prostheses and the simpler alternative of partial dentures is preferred.

The ability of a patient to afford treatment has a strong influence on the choice of restoration although the strength of this influence will vary with the contribution of any public funding to support the costs of treatment. An examination of the initial costs of treatment provision would suggest that partial dentures are the least costly treatment option. This undoubtedly contributes to their status as by far the most common means of replacing missing teeth. Such considerations tend to ignore the potential for long-term maintenance and additional treatment costs. Regrettably, a comparative cost benefit analysis of the various treatment options is lacking.

An interim replacement for missing teeth
Partial dentures may be required as an interim measure in a general treatment plan for the restoration of a partially edentulous mouth. They may aid the transition to edentulousness when the eventual loss of all remaining teeth and the use of complete dentures seem inevitable. These dentures are by

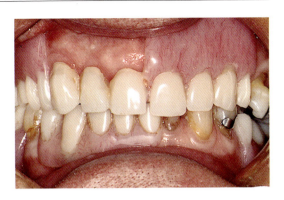

Fig 2-13 Overlay partial dentures used to restore occlusal face height and appearance for the patient illustrated in Fig 2-12b.

nature temporary and are termed transitional partial dentures. They are considered in more detail in Chapter 7.

Key Points

- Not all missing teeth need to be replaced. Their replacement should be based on a perceived patient need using a functionally oriented approach.
- A functionally oriented approach will result in reduced but more effective provision of partial dentures.
- Several factors influence the use of partial dentures. These include the nature of the edentulous space, the quality of potential abutment teeth, soft tissue loss and anterior tooth spacing, patient preference and cost.
- Other indications for partial dentures include their use as interim or transitional prostheses.

Further Reading

Jepson NJ, Allen PF. Short and sticky options in the treatment of the partially dentate patient. Br Dent J 1999;187:646–652.

Öwall B, Kayser AF, Carlsson GE. Prosthodontics: Principles and Management Strategies. St Louis, MO: Mosby, 1995.

Chapter 3
Basic Principles of Partial Denture Design

Aim

Partial dentures present clear advantages to both patient and clinician. However, partial denture designs that try to maximise these benefits also should attempt to minimise the potential for harm. This chapter aims to establish broad guidelines for the design of partial dentures that go some way in satisfying both these objectives.

Outcome

After reading this chapter, the practitioner should be aware of the principles of partial denture design that aim to maximise the functional stability of the denture and, at the same time, reduce the propensity of partial dentures to cause long-term harm to the remaining teeth and supporting soft tissues.

Classification of Partial Dentures

The part of the partial denture carrying the replacement teeth is called the "saddle". The natural teeth at the end of the saddle are termed "abutment" teeth. Where there is an abutment tooth at each end of the saddle it is termed a "bounded" saddle. Where there is no distal abutment tooth the saddle is described as "unbounded", distal extension or, more commonly, a free-end saddle. Saddles are typically made of acrylic and may be attached to a cast metal framework (definitive partial dentures that are designed for long-term use; Fig 3-1), or form a part of all acrylic dentures (transitional dentures intended for short-term use; Fig 3-2).

Given the huge number of possible permutations of both the number and distribution of missing teeth, it is not surprising that several attempts have been made to classify types of partial denture and relate these to particular designs. Whilst it is neither easy nor desirable to apply standard denture designs to individual cases, a classification does provide a convenient means of communication. Perhaps the best known and widely used is the Kennedy classification that is based on the relationship of the most posterior edentulous space to the remaining teeth (Box 3-1). Clinical examples of the

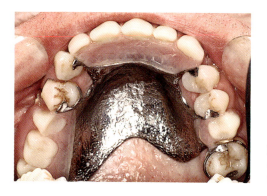

Fig 3-1 A partial denture with a cobalt-chromium metal framework.

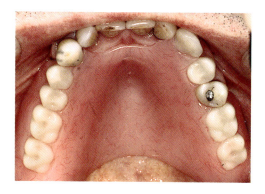

Fig 3-2 An all-acrylic, transitional partial denture.

Box 3-1

The Kennedy Classification for Partially Dentate Mouths

Class I   *Bilateral free-end saddles*
Class II   *Unilateral free-end saddle*
Class III   *Unilateral bounded saddle*
Class IV   *Saddle anterior to the standing teeth*

Classes I–III are subdivided into modifications, each modification denoting an additional saddle area.

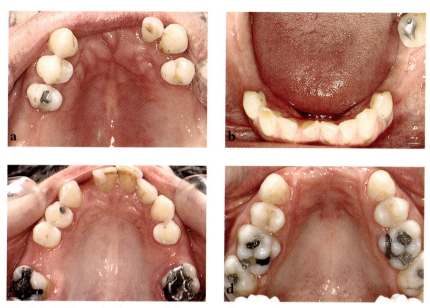

Fig 3-3 (a) Kennedy class I modification 1. (b) Kennedy class II modification 1. (c) Kennedy class III modification 2. (d) Kennedy class IV.

Kennedy classification, including some modifications, are illustrated in Fig 3-3.

Design and Stability in Function

For a partial denture to function effectively it is essential that the denture resists the forces that will try to displace it during use – meaning, it should have "stability in function". The major force acting on the denture is vertical loading during mastication and clenching with associated, but smaller, lateral forces. Pressure from the tongue, cheeks and lips will additionally tend to displace the denture laterally and anteroposteriorly during swallowing and speech. Finally, adherence of replacement teeth to the food bolus and gravity (in the upper jaw) will tend to displace the denture away from the tissues. Design features needed to ensure stability in function are summarised in Box 3-2.

The vertical loads of mastication and clenching are transmitted to the underlying bone via the hard and soft tissues on which the denture rests – the denture support. This may be tensile loading by way of the periodontal mem-

Box 3-2

Stability in Function: Summary of Design Criteria

Components giving adequate support, retention and bracing
Tooth support via rests when possible
Mucosally supported saddles should have wide extensions
Connectors, rests and bracing components must be rigid
Simultaneous bilateral occlusal contacts between natural or prosthetic teeth

branes of the remaining natural teeth (tooth support), compressive loading acting directly through the mucosa (mucosal support) or both, tooth and mucosal support (Fig 3-4). All partial dentures fall into one of these three categories. The ability of the supporting tissues to withstand masticatory loading increases with the area of available support. The greater the support, the more effective are the replacement teeth in penetrating the food bolus. The area of support offered by the healthy periodontium of a tooth is three to four times greater than that available from the residual ridge should that tooth be extracted. In addition, it is said that bone reacts more favourably to tensile rather than compressive loading. For these reasons tooth support should be used whenever possible.

When planning for tooth support, consideration should be given to the number and distribution of the denture teeth, the nature of the abutment teeth and the health of their periodontium. As a rule of thumb, an abutment can carry its own masticatory load plus that of one and a half replacement units. Canines and first and second molars provide good support whereas lower incisors and upper lateral incisors are likely to offer poor support, although this is modified in the light of past periodontal disease (Fig 3-5).

Where tooth support is considered inadequate then additional tissue support should be planned. When tissue support is used an attempt should be made to reduce the load acting on the tissues. This may be achieved by extending the fitting surface of the denture as widely as possible and by reducing the number or the width of the teeth on the denture (Fig 3-6). This is, of course, good prosthodontic practice as is applied in, and probably derived from, complete denture construction. Finally, if the replace-

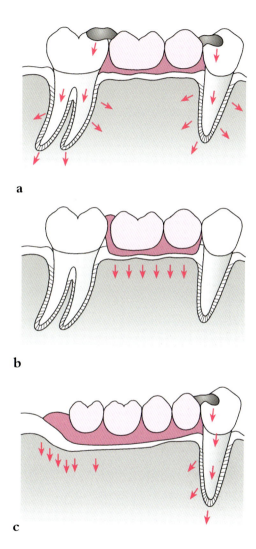

a

b

Fig 3-4 Types of available support for partial dentures. (a) Tooth support via rests illustrating the resulting tensile loading of the supporting bone as vertical loading is directed via the periodontal membrane. (b) Compressive loading of the underlying bone resulting from mucosal support of the denture saddle. (c) Combination of tooth and mucosal support seen in free-end saddle dentures.

c

ment teeth are to improve masticatory function it is necessary that they provide bilateral and simultaneous contact between natural and prosthetic teeth at an acceptable occlusal face height. For most patients this will coincide with an existing stable position of maximum intercuspation (Fig 3-7).

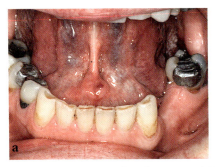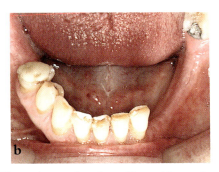

Fig 3-5 Assessment of tooth support. (a) The canines and molars will provide excellent potential tooth support for the bounded saddle. (b) The tilted molar and lateral incisor are unlikely to offer adequate tooth support for this long bounded saddle and this should be augmented by mucosal support. A combination of tooth and mucosal support is the best that can be achieved for the free-end saddle on the right.

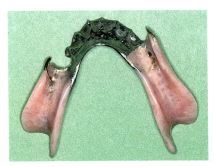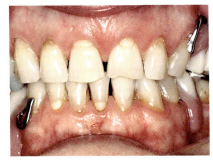

Fig 3-6 Use of the basic prosthodontic principle of broad extensions when mucosal support is required.

Fig 3-7 Occlusal contacts of partial dentures designed to coincide with and reinforce an existing intercuspal position.

Resistance to forces tending to displace the denture away from the tissues – denture retention – is dependent upon several factors. Of these, muscular control of the denture by the patient and the physical forces of adhesion and cohesion developed by the close adaptation of the fitting surface of the denture to the underlying tissues are common to all types of removable prosthesis. In the long-term, they are the significant factors for successful retention. However, for many partial dentures there is a need for further mechanical retention. This is provided by direct and indirect retainers. Direct retainers offer resistance to movement of the denture away from the tissues along its planned path of withdrawal. Indirect retainers act to prevent rotational displacement of the denture away from the tissues as, for example, in the free-end saddle denture.

How much retention is required of a given denture is difficult to define. It is presumably related to the size, number and type of saddles, i.e. longer saddles require more retention than shorter saddles, and bounded saddles less retention than free-end saddles. In addition, it is a common observation that retainers are ineffective after some years and yet the patient does not complain that the denture is loose (Fig 3-8). This emphasises the importance of the patient's muscular control in the long-term. Assuming their initial effectiveness, in practice there is rarely a need for more than two direct retainers.

Lateral displacing forces are said to be potentially the most damaging to the supporting structures of the teeth and the residual ridge and a wide distri-

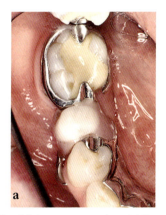
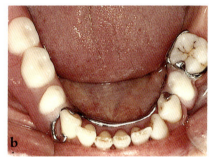

Fig 3-8 Partial denture retention. (a) Despite the ineffectiveness of the clasp on LR4 the patient had no complaint about the retention of the partial denture. (b) Two well-designed clasps will ensure adequate retention for this partial denture.

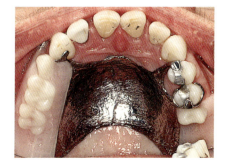

Fig 3-9 Minor connectors, clasp reciprocal arms, cingulum rest and flanges of the denture saddles will all contribute to bracing for this partial denture. Their effectiveness is ensured by the rigid palatal major connector.

bution of resistance is advised. This resistance is termed bracing. As with support, teeth offer the best resistance and tissues of the edentulous ridge or palate less so (Fig 3-9).

For components transmitting loads to teeth to act effectively, they must themselves be rigid and joined to the saddles and other components by rigid connectors.

Design and the Prevention of Harmful Effects

Clearly effective plaque control is the most important factor that prevents a long-term increase in the incidence of caries and periodontal disease. However, certain principles of design help minimise harmful effects. These are summarised in Box 3-3.

Box 3-3

Prevention of Harm: Summary of Design Criteria

Avoid unnecessary gingival coverage
Tooth support when gingivae are covered
Simplicity of design
Full extension of mucosally supported saddles

Gingival coverage, in particular, is associated with increased plaque formation and should be avoided whenever possible (Fig 3-10). Where this is not possible, then the part of the denture covering the gingiva should be tooth-supported and minimally relieved at the gingival sulcus. Failure to provide this support simply results in trauma to the underlying gingival tissues as the denture is displaced in function. Relief of the gingival margins without adequate tooth support results in the proliferation of gingival tissues into the space.

The design of the denture should be as simple as compatibility with function. Many partial denture components can be eliminated without endangering the rehabilitative functions of the denture (Fig 3-11). As discussed above, subjective clinical opinion suggests that well extended mucosally supported saddles tend to reduce resorptive changes.

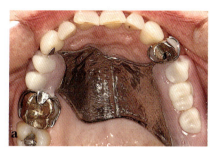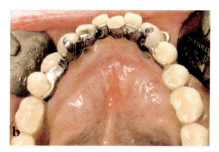

Fig 3-10 Examples of (a) an upper and (b) a lower partial denture where components have been designed to clear the gingival margin. (Courtesy of Prof. B. Öwall.)

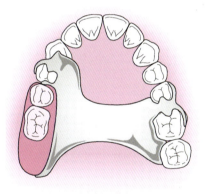

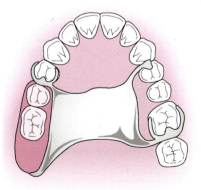

Fig 3-11 The simplification of design by
elimination of unnecessary components.

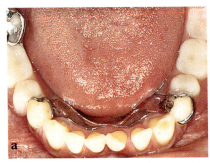 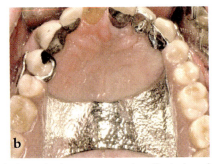

Fig 3-12 The application of current basic design criteria to a conventionally designed partial denture (a) and a "hygienic" partial denture design (b). (Courtesy of Prof. B. Öwall.)

Partial Denture Design: Current Principles

Traditionally, the design of partial dentures has focused on mechanisms to ensure adequate retention, stability and durability of the denture. Use of the several denture components deemed necessary to ensure stability in function is founded more on pragmatic clinical practice rather than a solid evidence base. Indeed, components of a partial denture required for stability in function may contribute to a long-term harmful effect for which there is a strong and growing evidence base. Current concepts of partial denture design attempt to address this potential conflict through the application of "hygienic principles". These emphasise the need for gingival clearance and simplicity through the use of the minimum number of components needed to ensure stability. Effective application of these principles generally requires a cast alloy framework and examples of such designs are illustrated in Fig 3-12. Both the functional and physical shortcomings of simple acrylic mucosal borne dentures preclude their use as anything but short-term, transitional partial dentures.

Key Points

Current design principles that address both the need for stability in function and the prevention of harm are:
• avoid unnecessary gingival coverage
• use tooth support whenever possible and wide extension of mucosally supported saddles
• use two retainers per denture
• use rigid connectors, rests and bracing components
• ensure simultaneous bilateral occlusal contacts between natural and/or prosthetic teeth.

Chapter 4
Partial Denture Design: Saddles, Rests and Retainers

Aim

This chapter will consider the design and function of the specific partial denture components – saddles, rests and retainers – in the context of the basic design principles for stability in function and the prevention of harm, and how these components can be incorporated into partial denture designs that follow "hygienic" principles. The particular problems of providing effective support and retention for free-end saddle partial dentures will also be considered.

Outcome

After reading this chapter the practitioner should be able to recognise the important design features of partial denture saddles, rests and retainers and understand how this design relates to the effective functioning of these partial denture components.

Saddles

The saddle is that part of the denture that rests on and covers the tissues of the alveolar ridge. It carries the artificial teeth and gum work. The design features of relevance are the:
• relationship of the saddle to the abutment tooth
• extension of the fitting surface of the saddle
• material of the fitting surface
• design of the occlusal surfaces.

Saddle–abutment relationship

There should normally be contact between the replacement tooth and the proximal surface of the abutment tooth to prevent food packing. Where possible, this contact should be with the natural contact area of the abutment tooth (Fig 4-1). Assuming that there is no aesthetic requirement for spacing between replacement and adjacent natural teeth.

The natural bulbosity or tilting of the abutment tooth often results in a space between the saddle and proximal surface of the abutment tooth. This area of unwanted undercut when enclosed by the denture is termed as dead space. Since it is claimed that these dead spaces predispose to food packing and perhaps increased plaque accumulation, they are undesirable. Two solutions to this supposed problem exist:

- Elimination of the dead space by altering the line of insertion of the denture or the shape of the abutment tooth – a closed saddle–abutment relationship (Fig 4-2a).
- Deliberate enlargement of the space and a reduction of the buccolingual width of the saddle next to the abutment tooth – an open saddle–abutment relationship (Fig 4-2b).

The latter approach better conforms to the requirement of avoiding gingival coverage and indeed there is evidence to suggest that this is more conducive to gingival health. However, spacing towards the front of the mouth may result in an unacceptable appearance. When a closed design is used, trauma to the gingival tissues can be prevented by providing both tooth support and slight relief of the gingival sulcus.

Extension of the fitting surface

Extension of the fitting surface is largely dependent upon the contribution the saddle is to make to the support of the denture. Where mucosal support is planned the design principle of maximum extension should be applied. This is clearly the case for simple mucosal borne dentures but applies equally to tooth/tissue supported free-end saddles (Fig 4-3).

The design of tooth-supported bounded saddles is less clear. When tooth support alone is adequate, as is often true of short posterior bounded sad-

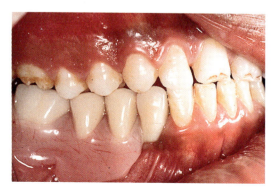

Fig 4-1 Contact of the replacement tooth established with the natural contact point of the abutment tooth.

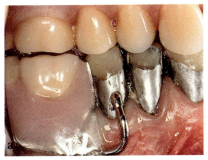 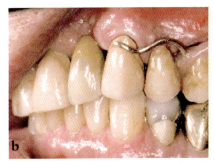

Fig 4-2 Closed (a) and open (b) saddle–abutment relationships. (Courtesy of Prof. B. Öwall.)

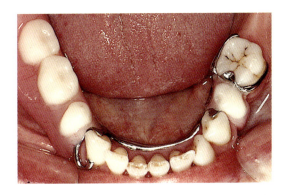

Fig 4-3 Broad extension of the free-end saddle. Extension of the short bounded saddle has been minimised.

dles, there is no need for broad mucosal coverage. A marked reduction in saddle size with an "open" saddle–abutment relationship offers the further advantages of increased freedom of movement for the tongue and cheeks, and avoidance of the gingival margin. Long bounded saddles and/or saddles with abutment teeth of poor support generally require additional tissue support and the maxim of wide extension again applies. In this context the buccal and lingual flanges may be important in resisting horizontal displacing forces by acting as bracing components.

The design of anterior saddles is normally dictated by aesthetic requirements. Dead spaces between replacement and adjacent teeth should be avoided and a "closed" design used. Where there has been considerable bone loss of the anterior edentulous ridge, a labial flange will be necessary to replace this loss and restore a normal appearance. In contrast, a labial flange where only slight resorption or a deep labial undercut is present will tend to result in an over-

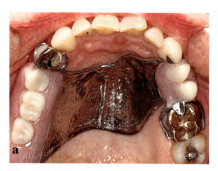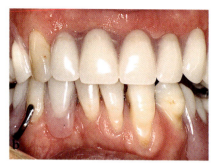

Fig 4-4 The design of anterior saddles. (a) A labial flange and a closed saddle–abutment relationship. (b) Minimal resorption and persistence of deep labial undercut preventing the use of a labial flange.

full lip and poor appearance (Fig 4-4). Such a decision will be made despite the undoubted functional advantages, i.e. resistance to backward and rotational displacing forces. When a labial flange is used, its extension need only be the amount necessary to ensure concealment of its upper edge by the lips.

Design of the occlusal surface

Replacement teeth should be positioned to allow bilateral, simultaneous contact with opposing teeth. When tissue support is planned, limiting the area of the occlusal table reduces the masticatory loads on the underlying tissue by improving the ease of penetration of the food bolus by the teeth. This is achieved by using narrow posterior teeth and reducing their number. This is of particular importance in the lower free-end saddle denture where it has the added advantage of providing more space for the tongue to control the denture (Fig 4-5).

Material of the fitting surface

The fitting surface of the saddle can be constructed in acrylic or metal. The advantage of acrylic is that it may be easily added to or modified and its use is advisable when further resorption of the alveolar ridge is expected. This is normally the case with free-end saddle dentures. The acrylic base is joined to the metal framework by way of a spaced meshwork cast as a part of the framework.

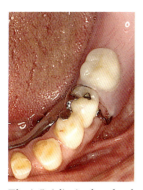

Fig 4-5 A limited occlusal table to reduce masticatory loads and allow space for control of the free-end saddle with the tongue.

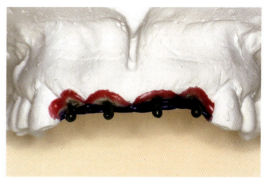

Fig 4-6 Studs to retain the replacement teeth positioned for the wax-up of a tissue fitting metal framework.

A metal base forms an integral part of cast metal framework and closely fits the supporting soft tissues. Its use leaves more space for the replacement teeth and this often results in better appearance anteriorly. The replacement teeth and associated gum work are retained on the metal base by means of retention tags or studs cast as a part of the framework. These are positioned to lie beneath and within the artificial teeth (Fig 4-6).

Rests

Tooth support through the use of rests should be used wherever possible. Rests are simply metal projections attached to the denture that extend onto the occlusal or prepared tooth surfaces. They are normally cast as a part of a metal framework. Rests may be placed upon sound enamel, or on direct or indirect restorations although the use of direct restorations is the least desirable because of their comparative weakness.

Rests serve to:

• transmit axial loads to a tooth
• deflect food away from the saddle–abutment tooth junction
• improve occlusal contacts when used as onlays
• act as indirect retainers and as auxiliary support for major connectors.

The ability of rests to transmit occlusal loads to the tooth is debatable. Findings that the mean clenched load on tooth–borne dentures is approximately half that on natural teeth suggest that they are not particularly effective. There is no convincing evidence to suggest that one design or position of a rest is more effective than any other. Clinical testing of such theories has been infrequent, contradictory and is possibly of limited clinical value. Pragmatically one simply uses the abutment teeth available, even severely periodontally weakened teeth can provide useful support. When this support is considered inadequate it should be augmented with additional tooth and/or mucosal support.

Design guidelines for rests are listed in Box 4-1. The requirements of, in particular, rigidity and conformity with the existing occlusion generally require preparation of the abutment tooth to create space for the rest. Even where space is not a problem, rest seat preparations give a clear indication to the technician of the intended position and extent of the rest.

There are several types of rest. Some examples are illustrated in Fig 4-7.

Box 4-1

Essential Features of Rests

Rigidity
Non-interference with existing intercuspal and lateral occlusion
Rounded to permit movement in function

Rests in posterior teeth – occlusal rests

The occlusal rest can be likened to a saucered spoon. It is broadest at the marginal ridge and tapers down into the adjacent fossa. The deepest part of the rest should form an angle of less than 90° with the vertical minor connector. This ensures positive seating of the rest. It should be of a thickness that ensures rigidity.

Rests in anterior teeth

Cingulum rests
These are designed to fit the prepared or augmented cingulum of usually a canine or maxillary incisor tooth. They may occupy the full width of the cingulum, its mesial or distal half or be confined to the marginal ridge when they are referred to as "marginal rests".

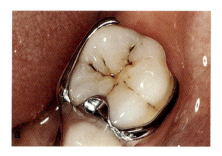 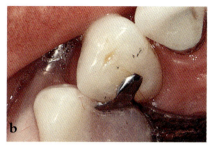

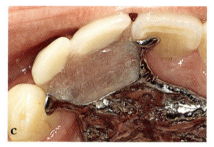 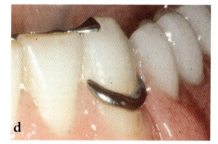

Fig 4-7 Rests: (a) occlusal, (b) cingulum, (c) marginal and (d) incisal.

Incisal rests

An incisal rest is used predominantly as an auxiliary rest or for indirect retention and is most frequently used on mandibular canines. It occupies a prepared rounded notch at an incisal angle with its deepest part directed towards the centre of the tooth. Aesthetically, incisal rests are the least desirable form of rest, in particular where the mesio-incisal angle is involved. Appearance can be improved if the rest is sited a short distance away from the incisal angle thus retaining some enamel between the rest and the mesio or disto-incisal angle. A modification of the incisal rest is the embrasure hook (or mesiodistal grip). This is a combination of mesial and distal incisal rests that extend onto the labial surface thereby providing some resistance to backward displacement of the denture.

Retainers

Retainers are components that prevent movement of the partial denture away from the tissues. They are described as "direct" when applied to abutment teeth to prevent withdrawal of the denture along its chosen path of insertion, or "indirect" when applied to teeth at a distance from a possible axis of rotation of a denture.

Direct retainers

Direct retainers may be further classified as extracoronal, of which the common example is the clasp, or intracoronal that usually take the form of precision attachments although there are examples of extracoronal precision attachments. Further discussion will be confined to extracoronal clasp assemblies and, in particular, will address three questions:

- What are the features of an effective clasp assembly?
- What factors can affect the retention of clasps?
- How many clasps are required?

Effective clasp assemblies

The essential element of a clasp is a flexible retentive clasp arm that is designed to lie against an undercut surface of a tooth. The flexibility simply allows the arm to pass over the maximum bulbosity of the tooth and into undercut.

Were this not so, the patient could not seat the denture. The seated denture will be retentive if the force required to flex the clasp arm back over the bulbosity of the tooth exceeds that acting to lift the denture away from the tissues. To ensure effectiveness all clasps must conform to the design criteria listed in Box 4-2.

Prosthodontic texts are replete with descriptions and classifications of the many possible designs of clasps. Use of such texts as a "recipe book" for clasp design is both frustrating and illogical. By applying the design criteria described in Box 4-2 to the distribution of usable undercut on individual teeth it will be possible to design effective clasp simply and logically. These may indeed resemble those in the recipe books but their design and application is much simpler (Fig 4-8).

A useful and descriptive classification is that of occlusally approaching and gingivally approaching clasp arms (Fig 4-9) although it should be emphasised that no clasp design has been shown to be more effective than any other. The most effective clasp will be the one nearest to the saddle and the design of clasps should be the simplest possible compatible with effectiveness. Clearance of the gingival margin is possible with occlusally approaching retentive clasp arms together with rigid arms rather than plates as reciprocal components. Where gingivally approaching clasp arms are to be used, a simple I-bar is preferred. This should

Box 4-2

Essential Design Criteria for Effective Clasp Assemblies

Flexible retentive clasp arm – *an arm of metal the end of which is flexible and lies against an undercut surface of a tooth*

Reciprocation – *rigid component(s) in contact with the opposite side of the tooth to the retentive clasp arm. This resists lateral forces applied to the tooth by the retentive clasp arm as it moves out of undercut and forces it to flex*

Encirclement – *involvement of more than half the circumference of the tooth to preclude movement of the tooth out of the confines of the clasp arms as stresses are applied*

Support – *a rest that prevents gingival displacement of the clasp assembly*

Passivity – *the retentive clasp arm should exert no pressure on the tooth until it is activated by movement of the denture in function or on its removal from the mouth*

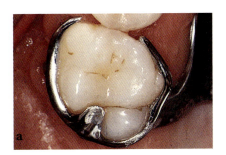
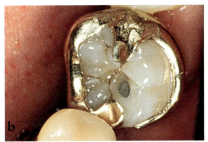
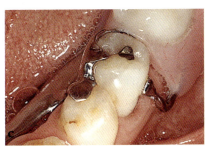
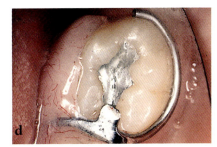

Fig 4-8 (a–d) Examples of widely differing designs of clasp all of which conform to the design criteria listed in *Box 4-2*. Passivity is assumed.

cross the gingival margin at a right angle and continue down for a further 2–3 mm before curving back into the saddle. The use of gingivally approaching clasps is contraindicated in the presence of deep soft tissue undercut. The retentive clasp arm cannot enter this undercut and their attempted use in these circumstances results in a space between the clasp arm and the tissues. This is likely to result in trauma to the adjacent buccal mucosa and will almost certainly act as a food trap.

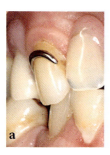 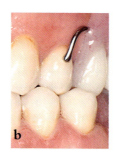

Fig 4-9 Examples of (a) occlusally and (b) gingivally approaching retentive clasp arms.

Factors affecting clasp retention
Excluding for the moment other important features influencing the retention of a denture, the amount of retention developed by a given clasp assembly depends upon several factors:

- Depth of undercut – This is really self-evident. For a given clasp, the greater the depth of undercut engaged the greater the resistance to withdrawal. The height and breadth of undercut area engaged will influence retention to a lesser extent.
- Mechanical properties of the alloy and dimensions of the retentive clasp arm The flexibility of the retentive clasp arm, i.e. how easily it can bend over the bulbosity of the tooth, will clearly affect retention. Both of the above factors have their principal effects on flexibility. The important mechanical properties are the modulus of elasticity, proportional limit and elongation. The modulus describes the stiffness of the alloy and its proportional limit the point beyond which further flexure results in permanent deformation. Elongation is a measure of how easily a clasp may be bent back after being permanently deformed. In broad terms the ideal alloy for clasps would have a low modulus of elasticity, a high proportional limit and high elongation. None of the commonly used alloys fulfils these criteria, the best probably being gold alloy.
- For a given alloy, flexibility will vary with the dimension and shape of the

retentive clasp arm. The important variables are thickness, length and curvature. A reduction in thickness by half will increase flexibility eight-fold. Doubling the length of the retentive clasp arm will again increase flexibility eight-fold. The tighter the curvature the more rigid the clasp.

- Clasp design – It is possible to vary the retention of a clasp by altering the depth of engaged undercut and its size and shape. In practice, the length and curvature of the retentive clasp arm is restricted by the shape of the tooth and, perhaps more significantly, by the position of the undercut on the tooth to be clasped. Variations in flexibility are, therefore, limited in practice to changing the alloy or clasp thickness. Use of this change in thickness to improve flexibility is clearly seen in the design of a cobalt-chromium retentive clasp arm. Here the use of a tapered pattern with this stiff alloy allows an improved flexibility of the terminal half of the retentive clasp arm (Fig 4-10). As a general guide, when cobalt-chromium alloys are used the clasps should be of adequate length (15 mm), minimum curvature and engage an undercut of 0.25 mm.

- The mobility of clasped teeth – If the reciprocating component does not remain in contact with the tooth as the denture is displaced away from the tissues – this may often be the case – the retentive clasp arm is free to apply a force laterally to the tooth. The clasp essentially moves out of the undercut and will no longer be effective. The load required to move a normally supported tooth about 0.1 mm is said to be as low as 100g and this will reduce as tooth mobility increases. Such tooth movement under limited loading should be taken into account when planning with the 0.25 mm depth of undercut normally engaged by a cobalt-chromium clasp arm. A suggested force of some 1.5 kg required to retain a free-end saddle denture does emphasise the limitations of clasp retention in this situation.

Fig 4-10 Use of a tapered pattern for the terminal half of a cobalt-chromium retentive clasp arm to improve its flexibility as it passes into the undercut. All other parts of the clasp are rigid and placed on or above the survey line.

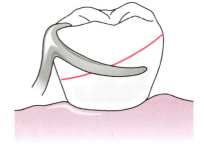

The number of clasps required
The recommendation that only two direct retainers are used is based on subjective clinical experience. Clasps are not the only means of retention because effective retention can be gained by engaging proximal, buccal and labial undercut with the rigid material of the saddle. Furthermore, factors such as adhesion and cohesion, polished surface shape and muscular activity assume greater importance with time, although their contribution will depend upon the number, size and type of saddles.

Support and retention of free-end saddle dentures
Differential support
The absence of a distal abutment tooth reduces the support available to a free-end saddle denture and the best that can be achieved is a combination of tooth and mucosal support. In this case, when masticatory load is applied to the saddle the rest seat will limit movement mesially to a very slight depression of the abutment tooth within its periodontal ligament. However, because of the greater displaceability of the soft tissues, the posterior part of the saddle will tend to sink further – "differential displacement" that results in the denture rotating about the occlusal rest. It should be noted that such displacement does not usually occur in the upper arch since the major connector will usually be supported by the typically firm tissues of the midline of the hard palate.

Rotation
The likely rotation of the free-end saddle denture about the occlusal rest when masticatory loads are applied will result in the anterior part of the framework lifting away from the teeth. This instability in function is assumed to affect the comfort and efficiency of the denture and has been shown *in vivo* to result in an uneven distribution of load both to the abutment tooth and to the supporting tissues of the denture base with the load concentrated distal to the abutment tooth and beneath the distal end of the denture base.

Clasp design
The design of clasps for free-end saddle dentures should follow the guidelines indicated earlier in this chapter but their effectiveness will often be a compromise between the large retentive forces required of, in particular, Kennedy class I partial dentures and the practical limits on clasp retention imposed by the abutment teeth which are commonly premolars or canines. There are many theoretical considerations of clasp design for free-end saddle partial dentures. Most address the possibility of the clasp applying torque to the abutment tooth as the free-end saddle is depressed under masticatory load-

ing. Suggested solutions include increasing the flexibility of the retentive clasp arm by using wrought gold and the use of gingivally approaching clasps.

Rest position

Rest position and clasp design are said to influence the stress or torque applied to the abutment tooth in response to masticatory loads. In particular, an abutment tooth will be moved towards the side on which the rest is located. Rotation of the denture about a distal rest exerts forces on the abutment tooth that are said to result in its distal movement and increased mobility and, by concentrating stress at the distal end of the denture base, increased bone loss at the edentulous ridge (Fig 4-11). By transferring the occlusal rest to the mesial surface the resultant forces will tend to move the abutment tooth mesially. Further, by moving the axis of rotation to the mesial surface the arc of movement of the denture base is more perpendicular to the supporting soft tissues resulting in a more normal loading of the underlying mucosa. The RPI clasp design (mesial rest; proximal plate and gingivally approaching I-bar) was introduced specifically to address these supposed problems of unfavourable patterns of stress distribution to the abutment tooth and the tissues supporting the free-end saddle (Fig 4-12).

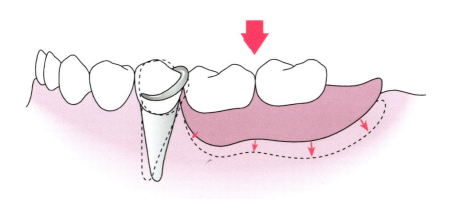

Fig 4-11 Differential displacement of a free-end saddle under masticatory load. A distal rest leads to stress concentration distal to the abutment tooth and at the distal end of the saddle. Rotation about the distal rest causes the clasp to grip the abutment tooth and displace it distally.

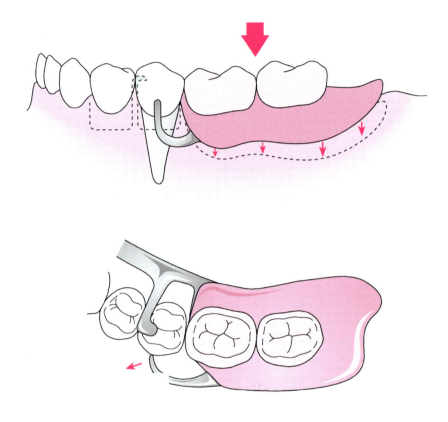

Fig 4-12 The RPI (rest, plate, I-bar) clasp is designed to ensure rotation about a mesial rest. This is said to reduce stress on the abutment tooth during masticatory loading as the clasp moves out of contact with the tooth and results in a more even distribution of stress beneath the free-end saddle.

The evidence base supporting these effects of rest placement and clasp design is weak but does suggest that:

- mesial placement of the occlusal rest, regardless of clasp design, results in reduced loading and improved stress distribution to the abutment tooth
- masticatory loads result in a forward movement of the denture base regardless of rest position or clasp design.

A more practical and effective approach is to reduce the potential for differential displacement in the first place. This is simply achieved using a displacement impression technique that records the soft tissues under load such that the processed free-end denture saddle will displace the tissues when seated and thus limit the potential movement of the denture base under occlusal load. Practical aspects of this technique are described under "Altered cast impression" in Chapter 11.

Indirect retainers

Despite the presence of direct retainers, rotational displacement of parts of the denture remote from the direct retainer is still possible. This is commonly seen with the free-end saddle denture. Here, the displacement occurs as a rotation of the saddles away from the tissues about a fulcrum drawn through the tips of the clasps on the abutment teeth, the clasp axis. It is prevented by providing indirect retention (Fig 4-13).

This is achieved by incorporating rigid components that contact teeth forward of the clasp tips. When the saddle now rotates away from the tissues, these new contacts will act as the fulcrum. The clasp is positioned between the new fulcrum and the free-end saddle and will resist its rotational displacement. The further these rigid components are placed away from the clasp axis the greater is the mechanical leverage acting against the rotational displacement of the saddle. Somewhat confusingly, the components effecting this forward positioning of this axis of rotation are termed indirect retainers. It should, however, be clear that there can be no indirect retention without effective direct retainers. Rests are the obvious and perhaps most effective examples of indirect retainers. Others include major connectors such as a lingual plate, lingual bar with continuous clasp and a modified continuous clasp (dental bar). These components are described in the following chapter.

There is no good evidence supporting the clinical effectiveness of indirect retainers which introduce additional gingival coverage and complicate the design of a partial denture. Despite this the use of indirect retainers with free-end saddle dentures is almost universally recommended by standard prostho-

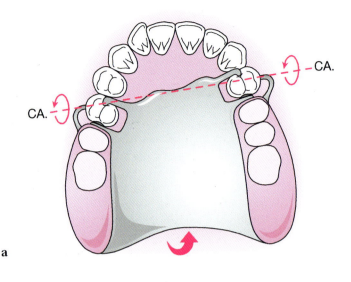

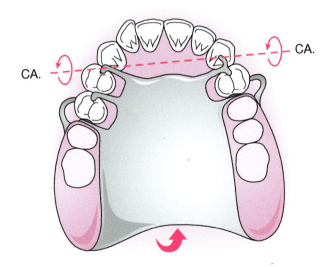

Fig 4-13 Providing indirect retention. (a) There is nothing to prevent rotation of the saddles away from the tissues about the clasp axis (CA). (b) The saddles now rotate about an axis between the rest seats placed on UR4 and UL3. The direct retainers at UR5 and UL4 placed between the new fulcrum and the saddles can now resist the rotatory displacement of the saddles.

dontic texts. This may reflect their role in facilitating the stabilisation of a metal framework when a reline impression is made.

Key Points

- Important features of partial denture saddles include the design of the occlusal surface, the relationship of the saddle to the abutment tooth, the extension of the fitting surface and the material used for its construction.
- Effective rests are rigid, conform to the existing occlusion and permit limited movement of the partial denture in function.
- All clasp designs should be based upon certain basic criteria. The retention offered by individual clasps is largely dictated by the morphology and periodontal status of the clasped tooth.
- A practical approach to the difficulty of ensuring adequate support and retention for lower free-end saddle partial dentures includes the use of a mesial rest on abutment teeth, effective clasps of conventional design and a displacement impression technique.
- Indirect retention is recommended for free-end saddle dentures but not at the expense of a overly complicated partial denture design.

Chapter 5
Partial Denture Design: Connectors

Aim

This chapter will consider the design and function of partial denture connectors in the context of the basic design principles of stability in function and for the prevention of harm. It will also aim to help the practitioner understand how these components can be incorporated into partial denture designs that follow "hygienic" principles.

Outcome

After reading this chapter the practitioner should be able to recognise the important design features of major connectors used for upper and lower partial dentures and the clinical factors that influence the selection of major connectors.

Introduction

The saddles and other components of the partial denture are joined by connectors. "Major" connectors link the saddles to the denture and "minor" connectors join components such as rests and clasps to the saddle and the major connector.

Major Connectors

General principles of design
The essential design requirements for major connectors are listed in Box 5-1. Major connectors should be rigid since it is only through this rigidity that all other components of the partial denture can be effective (the only exception to this rule is when flexible, stress-broken designs are deliberately used). Rigidity is a function of the length, width (height) and thickness of the connector, plates tending to be thin and wide, bars narrower but thicker. Rigidity dictates that no part of a major connector may enter an undercut and all unwanted undercuts in relation to the major connector must be blocked out prior to its construction.

Box 5-1

Essential Features of Major Connectors

Rigidity
Clearance of the gingival margin if possible
Minimal relief of the gingival sulcus if covered
Non-interference with movement of soft tissue
Support from components other than saddles

Coverage of the gingival margin should be kept to a minimum. The major connector should finish interproximally and where it is designed to be free of the gingival margin a clearance of at least 3 mm is recommended. Coverage of palatal and lingual surfaces is suggested when:

• There is insufficient space for a rigid connector with adequate clearance of the gingival margin.

• Additional support, bracing and indirect retention is required in an arch in which few natural teeth remain.

• The future loss of teeth is anticipated; coverage of palatal or lingual surfaces will simplify the addition of replacement teeth to the existing denture.

• There are several single tooth saddles to be connected. The attempt to clear the gingival margin in this circumstance often results in a complicated outline of the major connector that is uncomfortable for the patient, likely to encourage food trapping and can be difficult to cast accurately.

Minimal relief of the gingival sulcus should be provided when the connector covers the gingival margin. Inclusion of more substantial relief simply results in proliferation of the gingival tissues into the space.

Connectors should not prevent normal soft tissue movements or impinge on soft tissue when they move in function. Additional tissue relief is therefore normally indicated in anticipation of settling and rotation during function. Such relief is essential over inoperable tori, other exostoses, and prominent median palatal suture areas. The amount of relief is dependent upon the quality of support and resistance to rotation afforded by other components. It is, for example, likely that a free-end saddle denture will move more than a well retained and supported bounded saddle dentures.

All major connectors should be supported by components other than the saddles. This support is primarily derived from rests terminating in seats specifically prepared to receive them.

Maxillary major connectors

The broad extent of the palatal tissues available for the placement of the maxillary major connector means that availability of space is not normally a constraint on the use of rigid maxillary major connectors that avoid gingival coverage. More important factors that influence and constrain the design of maxillary major connectors include the number and distribution of edentulous spaces, the quality of the available denture support, palatal anatomical features and patient acceptance. The latter is better achieved by restricting the connector outline to the middle and/or posterior parts of the hard palate. Involvement of the more richly innervated anterior palatal tissues can be associated with greater patient intolerance and discomfort. In contrast, a gag reflex in a patient will prevent normal posterior extension of the upper connector. Some common examples of upper major connectors are described below.

Palatal plates

These take the form of broad straps or plates that serve effectively to unite bilateral saddles (Fig 5-1). Rigidity is not a problem and clearance of the gingival margin is readily achieved by ending the connector interproximally. The connector outline simply reflects the length and position of the denture saddles. As a general rule, the width of the connector across the palate should approximate that of the longest saddle. The position of the posterior border of the connector reflects the position of the most posterior saddle although its outline across the palatal midline will be influenced by the need for additional support and patient tolerance. The outline of the anterior border should normally follow and blend with the irregularities of the palatal rugae but, in the special circumstance of extensive bilateral free-end saddles, a decision may be made to extend the connector on to the palatal surfaces of the remaining anterior teeth. This can give better support and bracing and will introduce effective indirect retention. However, it is associated with gingival coverage. A more "hygienic" alternative would be a dental bar. A cast metal palatal connector that covers most of the hard palatal can lead to problems of denture retention simply through the weight of the connector. An alternative in this circumstance is to combine cast metal anterior elements with acrylic through the use of retentive loops incorporated into the metal part of the connector.

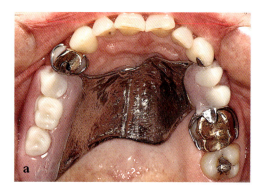

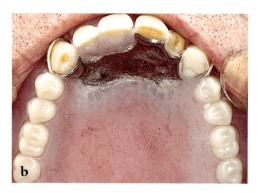

Fig 5-1 Maxillary plate type connectors. (a) The width of the mid-palatal strap across the palate reflects the length of the longest saddle. (b) The posterior extent of the connector and its extension on to the palatal surfaces of the few remaining anterior teeth reflects the need to improve support and bracing. The combination of metal anteriorly and acrylic posteriorly reduces the weight of the connector.

Anterior and posterior bars (ring connector)
The combination of anterior and posterior bars allows sufficient rigidity without recourse to more extensive palatal coverage (Fig 5-2). The use of this design is possible when tooth support is adequate and the quality of the soft tissue support for long bounded or free-end saddles is excellent. It can also be used when a prominent midline palatal torus prevents the use of a mid-palatal plate and the posterior element of the ring connector can be placed posterior to the palatal torus. The reduced coverage of the palatal tissues associated with this design is often preferred by patients as it improves appreciation of the texture of food. This may lead to difficulties in patients' acceptance when attempting to replace an inadequately supported ring connector with a design involving more extensive palatal coverage.

Horse-shoe connector
The name of this connector simply reflects its outline (Fig 5-3). It is perhaps

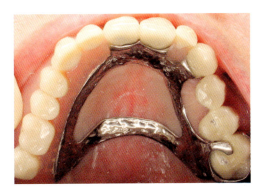

Fig 5-2 A ring connector.

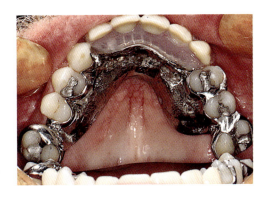

Fig 5-3 A horseshoe connector. Unfortunately, this connector is often associated with gingival coverage.

the least desirable design of upper major connector as it is often difficult to combine adequate rigidity with clearance of the gingival margin. This connector is indicated when a large palatal torus prevents placement of the connector in the mid and posterior palatal regions or when patients cannot tolerate the posterior extension of the upper connector.

Mandibular major connectors
Given the principal design objective of rigidity and gingival clearance, the main factor influencing the choice of lower major connector is the space available between the lingual gingival margin and the functional depth of the floor of the mouth anteriorly. In addition, as a consequence of the anatomical form of the anterior lingual soft tissues, lower major connectors can offer no additional mucosal support although some designs will contribute to indirect retention through their contact with the lingual surfaces of lower anterior teeth. Several distinct designs of lower major connector are described

and these essentially reflect the desire to use the principle of "hygienic" designs and the space available. These connector types and the clinical indications for their use are summarised in Table 5-1.

Table 5-1 **Clinical factors influencing the selection of lower major connectors**

Clinical factor	Lower major connectors				
	Lingual bar	Sublingual bar	Lingual plate	Dental bar	Buccal bar
Adequate space*	✓	✓	✗	✗	✗
Inadequate space	✗	✗	✓	✓	✗
Prominent lingual fraenum	?	✗	✓	✓	✗
Gingival recession	✗	✓	✗	✓	✗
Tooth spacing	✓	✓	?	?	✗
Short clinical crowns	✓	✓	✓	✗	✗
Poor prognosis of remaining teeth	✗	✗	✓	✗	✗
Lingual interferences	✗	✗	✗	✗	✓
Need for indirect retention	✗	✗	✓	✓	✗

*Adequate space means approximately 6–7 mm between the lingual gingival margin and the functional depth of the anterior lingual sulcus.

Lingual bar

The lingual bar is commonly described as the first choice for lower connectors that attempt to clear the gingival margin. In cross-section, the lingual bar should resemble a tear-drop with the greatest thickness at its lower margin that then reduces vertically as it approaches the upper margin in contact with the lingual soft tissues (Fig 5-4). To ensure rigidity the lingual bar should be approximately 3–4 mm high although this requirement will increase with the length of the bar. To ensure adequate clearance, the upper border should

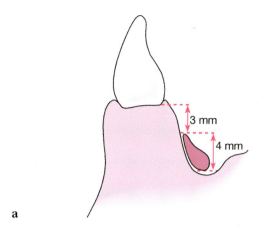

a

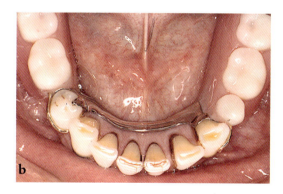

Fig 5-4 The lingual bar. (a) Dimensions and space requirements for a lingual bar. (b) Clinical appearance.

b

be placed 3 mm below the gingival margin and the lower border should be placed as far into the anterior lingual sulcus as functional movement of these tissues will allow. This effectively means a space requirement of about 6–7 mm between the slightly elevated lingual sulcus and the gingival margin. Gingival recession and a prominent lingual fraenum can reduce the available space and are common contraindications to the use of a lingual bar.

Sublingual bar

The sublingual bar was originally developed to address the problem of the relative flexibility of the lingual bar. It is designed to occupy the full functional depth and width of the anterior lingual sulcus (Fig 5-5). The result is a significant increase in thickness and therefore rigidity as compared to the lingual bar. In addition, the height of the sublingual bar is less than the lingual bar and this places the upper border of the bar further away from the gingival margin. This allows the use of the sublingual bar with adequate gingival clearance in the presence of gingival recession although a prominent lingual fraenum will still prevent its use. Food trapping can be associated with the use of the sublingual bar, in particular when there is tight contact of the superior border of the bar with the soft tissues. This can be reduced by introducing slight clearance between the sublingual bar and the underlying mucosa.

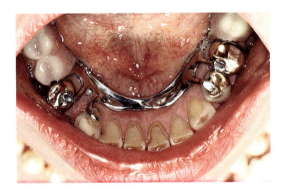

Fig 5-5 The sublingual bar occupying the functional anterior lingual sulcus with resulting increase in thickness.

Fabrication of the sublingual bar requires a controlled and accurate impression of the functional anterior lingual sulcus. Although this can complicate the impression procedures for a partial denture, the resultant cast provides the laboratory with a very clear prescription for the design of the major connector to the technician. In contrast and perhaps less desirably, construction of a lingual bar relies on the use of preformed wax patterns and the technician's discretion. The relative bulk of the sublingual bar suggests that patient tolerance of this connector may be problematic. However, a combination of the patient's awareness of its advantages and the relative lack of sensory perception in this region of the mouth normally results in good patient acceptance.

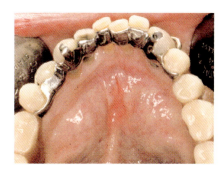

Fig 5-6 A dental bar. (Courtesy of Prof. B. Öwall.)

Dental bar / Kennedy Bar

The dental bar is a "hygienic" alternative when the lack of space or a prominent lingual fraenum prevents the use of a lingual or sublingual bar (Fig 5-6). It is indicated, in particular, in patients with gingival recession following periodontal treatment where clearance of the gingival margin will facilitate future plaque control. The outline of the dental bar follows that of the lingual coronal contour with thickening interproximally to ensure rigidity although this can result in reduced patient tolerance. Spacing between the remaining lower anterior teeth prevents the use of a dental bar unless the spacing is closed simply with adhesive composite restorations.

Lingual plate

The lingual plate is a frequently used alternative when space and anatomic limitations prevent the use of a lingual or sublingual bar (Fig 5-7). The outline of the lingual plate consists of a lingual bar which continues superiorly as an upper "apron" shaped to follow the lingual contours of the remaining

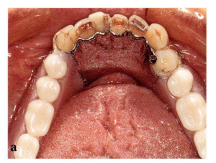 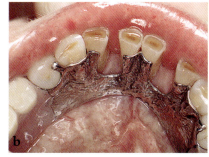

Fig 5-7 (a) Appearance of a conventional lingual plate. (b) Lingual plate cut away to accommodate spacing between anterior teeth.

anterior teeth. The lower border is positioned at the reflection of the functional lingual sulcus with the upper border ending at or on the cingulae of the lower anterior teeth. The major disadvantage of the lingual plate is the involved gingival coverage and its use is not recommended where the future maintenance of high levels of plaque control is essential to ensure the continuing periodontal health of the remaining teeth as will often be the case after successful periodontal therapy. The increased interproximal spacing often consequent to periodontal therapy will in any event result in an unacceptable show of metal should a lingual plate be used. The lingual plate is commonly used for severely shortened lower dental arches where it is said to augment available support and bracing and provide effective indirect retention. In particular, the lingual plate is indicated when some remaining teeth are of doubtful prognosis as the future addition of teeth to the lingual plate of an existing denture is a relatively straightforward procedure. Slight spacing between remaining anterior teeth can be accommodated by notching the upper apron of the lingual plate (see Fig 5-7b).

Buccal bar
The buccal bar is the last resort when severe lingual interferences – for example, lingually tilted teeth or inoperable mandibular tori, prevent the use of a lingual major connector or other restorative options for the replacement of the missing teeth (Fig 5-8). The presence of labial soft tissue undercut and the relative flexibility of the buccal bar resulting from its increased length compared with a lingual bar frequently cause difficulties in construction.

Kennedy bar (continuous clasp)
The Kennedy bar essentially combines a lingual bar and a continuous clasp and was used when space limitations prevented the construction of a rigid conventional lingual bar. The combination of a lingual bar of reduced thick-

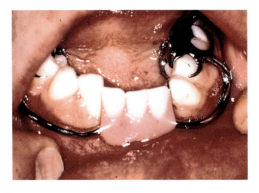

Fig 5-8 Use of a buccal bar where interferences presented by the severely lingually tilted posterior teeth prevent the use of any other connector.

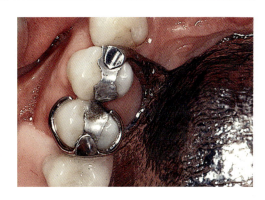

Fig 5-9 A minor connector linking the occlusal rest at UL4 to the major connector.

ness together with the continuous clasp ensured adequate rigidity of the connector. The difficulty is that the limitation of available space enforces the use of a smaller lingual bar resulting in the bar being place too close to the gingival margin. In addition, the continuous clasp that takes the form of a relatively thick, scalloped bar on the lingual surfaces of the teeth is frequently poorly tolerated by patients. There are more effective options to this connector, whose use should be considered as historic.

Minor Connectors

The design principle of rigidity applies equally to minor connectors. When joining rests and clasps to major connectors, minimal gingival coverage is achieved by placing the minor connector interproximally (Fig 5-9). Here, it should be triangular in form so as to fit the embrasure and occupy minimal space compatible with rigidity. The gingival margin should be crossed at a right angle and the junction with the major connector should be rounded rather than angular to prevent stress concentration within the framework casting.

Key Points

- Partial denture connectors should be rigid and avoid gingival coverage where this is possible.
- Upper major connectors may be palatal plates, anterior and posterior bars, or of the horse-shoe type.
- Upper connectors that are both rigid and avoid gingival coverage are normally easily achievable and factors such as the number, size and distribution of partial denture saddles, anatomical considerations and patients' tolerance are more important influences on upper major connector design.

- The important lower major connector designs are the lingual, buccal, sublingual and dental bars, and lingual plate.
- The availability of space is the major factor influencing the choice of lower major connectors that are both rigid and attempt to avoid gingival coverage. Additional factors pertain to the prognosis of the remaining teeth, their morphology and the anatomy of the associated soft tissues.

Chapter 6
Surveying

Aim

The aim of this chapter is to emphasise the essential role of the dental surveyor in the design process of partial dentures.

Outcome

After reading this chapter, the practitioner should understand the use of a dental surveyor to determine the path of insertion of a partial denture and be aware of the factors that influence the choice of the path of insertion.

Introduction

The basic principles of partial denture design were considered in Chapter 3 under the broad headings of "stability in function" and "prevention of harm". In more practical terms, the objective should be a finalised design that will allow the denture to:

- be easily inserted and removed by the patient
- resist dislodging forces
- be aesthetically pleasing
- avoid the creation of undesirable food traps
- minimise plaque retention.

This objective is achieved by a careful evaluation of a patient's study casts. The instrument used to aid the examination of the study cast is called a "surveyor" and the procedure is known as "surveying".

Surveying

The surveyor essentially comprises a vertical rod that is held perpendicular to a horizontal platform (Fig 6-1). The rod may be moved horizontally and up and down. Attached to the horizontal platform is the cast table to which the study cast is fastened. This may be positioned in various planes. The vertical rod represents the path along which the denture is inserted and removed

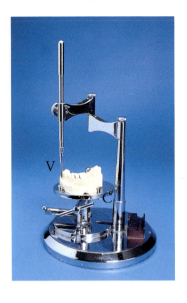

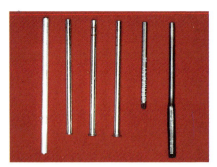

Fig 6-1 (left) A dental surveyor. The vertical rod (V) represents the path of insertion which can be changed by altering the tilt of the cast on the adjustable cast table (C).

Fig 6-2 (top) Surveyor tools (from left to right): analysing rod, 0.25, 0.5 and 0.75 undercut gauges, surveying lead, wax chisel.

– the path of insertion – and this can be altered by changing the tilt of the cast on the cast table. By positioning this vertical rod against the teeth and soft tissue areas of the cast, their morphology can be examined in relation to various paths of insertion. The various surveyor tools are illustrated in Fig 6-2.

For any given path of insertion, the contour line formed by joining points of maximum bulbosity on the teeth or soft tissues is termed the "survey line". Areas below the survey line are said to be undercut for that path of insertion. By placing a lead marker against the tooth or soft tissue, it should be possible to plot a high and low survey line for each undercut area. These should eventually join up and thus outline the entire undercut area (Fig 6-3). Any rigid part of the partial denture must be designed to lie outside of the surveyed undercut area and only flexible parts may be designed to go into it. The only flexible part of a partial denture is the terminal part of a retentive clasp arm.

Survey lines and associated undercut areas exist relative to a given path of insertion. Changing the path of insertion changes the survey line and undercut distribution (Fig 6-4). The final design should ideally permit a single precise path of insertion that is precisely determined by a consideration of the factors illustrated in Fig 6-5. Once the path of insertion has been decided

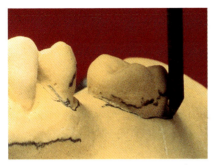 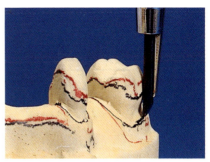

Fig 6-3 Upper and lower survey lines mapping the undercut area on the buccal surface of the molar.

Fig 6-4 The change in survey lines and undercut distribution for the path of natural displacement (red) and the chosen path of insertion (black).

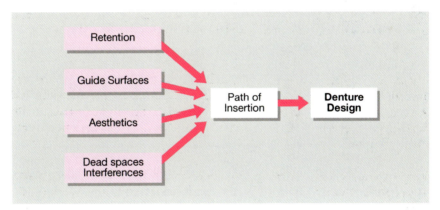

Fig 6-5 Factors influencing the choice of the path of insertion. Once this has been determined the design of the denture can be completed.

upon, the final design of the prosthesis can be completed. In practice the path of insertion frequently has to be a compromise between these often conflicting factors.

Retention
All dentures will tend to move away from the supporting tissues during function. This is largely because of adherence of the denture teeth to food during mastication and additionally, in the upper, to the effects of gravity. For an individual partial denture this displacement may be possible in several directions. However, it is generally assumed that all partial dentures will have

a tendency to withdraw along a path at right angles to the occlusal plane – the "path of natural displacement". If the partial denture is to be retentive then resistance to this natural displacement must be provided. This is achieved by engaging retentive undercut that exists relative to the path of natural displacement with either clasps or rigid parts of the denture in one of the following three ways:

- With clasps using a path of insertion at right angles to the occlusal plane, i.e. similar to the path of natural displacement (Fig 6-6). In this case, retention is contingent upon the effectiveness of the clasps alone. The use of "open" saddle–abutment relationships in the posterior bounded partial denture dictates this approach.

- By selecting a path of insertion that is clearly not at right angles to the occlusal plane (Fig 6-7). Using this approach, rigid parts of the denture can be placed in areas which are undercut relative to natural displacement. One example is the free-end saddle denture in which resistance to natural displacement is provided by the saddle engaging undercut distal to the abutment tooth. This normally results in a "closed" saddle–abutment relationship. Reasonably one would expect a rigid component to provide more resistance to natural displacement than a flexible retentive clasp arm. In practical terms, however, the success of this approach is very much dependent upon the use of effective guide surfaces to restrict and reinforce the chosen path of insertion (see Guide surfaces later).

- A combination of both of the above approaches. This is perhaps the most effective way of ensuring retention. A good example is partial dentures replacing anterior teeth (Fig 6-8). A path of insertion is chosen that reduces labial undercut and allows seating of the rigid labial flange. This area is undercut relative to the path of natural displacement. Clasps on posterior teeth are then designed to engage undercut common to both the planned path of insertion and the path of natural displacement.

In summary, if there is a good reason to choose a path of insertion that differs from the path of natural displacement, clasps should be designed to engage undercut relative to both paths of withdrawal. If retentive undercut for clasps is available and there is no other reason to alter the path of insertion, use of the path of natural displacement as the path of insertion is perfectly acceptable. The chosen path of insertion does not have to differ from that of natural displacement.

Ideally the clasp undercuts should be equally distributed, that is they should not be very deep on some abutment teeth and very shallow on others, but this cannot always be achieved. Only minor modifications to the

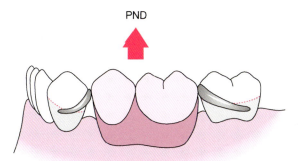

Fig 6-6 Retention using clasps engaging undercut present for the path of natural displacement (PND).

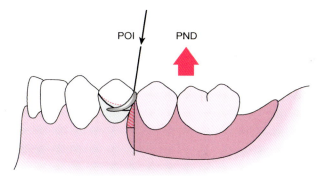

Fig 6-7 By altering the path of insertion (POI) rigid parts of the denture (in this case the saddle acrylic) can engage areas of the proximal surface that are undercut relative to the path of natural displacement (PND).

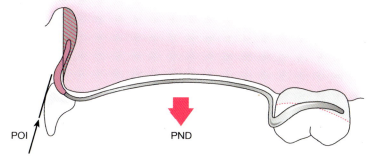

Fig 6-8 Choosing the illustrated path of insertion (POI) allows placement of a rigid labial flange in areas undercut relative to the path of natural displacement (PND). The clasps on molar teeth are then designed to engage undercut common to both the POI and PND.

path of insertion should be made to improve these undercuts. Where little or no clasp undercut exists for an otherwise reasonable path of insertion, it is usually preferable to create undercuts by restorative means rather than to compromise the path of insertion. The final design of the clasps must always be deferred until the retentive undercut distribution has been revealed.

Guide surfaces (guiding planes)

Guide surfaces are a series of surfaces parallel to each other and the path of insertion that ensure that the dentures can be inserted or withdrawn along the selected path of insertion (Fig 6-9). To be effective they should be at least 2–3 mm long. The restricted path of insertion and withdrawal has in theory several advantages:

- Improved clasp function – It should always be remembered that an undercut exists only in relation to the chosen path of insertion and withdrawal. If the denture can be displaced along another path there may be no undercut relative to this other path and effective retention is illusory. A restricted path of withdrawal therefore ensures the predictability of the planned retentive undercut. Further, when reciprocal clasp arms or plates contact guide surfaces their contact against the tooth is maintained as the denture moves away from the tissues. Effective reciprocation is maintained and the flexible retentive clasp arm must flex if it is to withdraw from undercut. Finally, a restricted path of insertion prevents the possible distortion of the flexible retentive clasp arm that can occur if another path of insertion could be used to seat the denture.
- Ease of insertion and removal of the denture by the patient.
- Frictional contact of denture components against guide surfaces may assist the overall retention of the partial denture.
- Reduction of dead space – The management of dead spaces is described in more detail later in this chapter.

The perfect example of a guide surface is a precision attachment. Next in order of effectiveness are prepared parallel surfaces incorporated into cast coronal restorations on abutment teeth where extensive restoration is required (Fig 6-10). Guide surfaces also may be prepared by grinding the surface enamel of abutment teeth although the chances of creating several tooth surfaces that are parallel to each other and the path of insertion are limited (see Chapter 10). In the absence of restoration or preparation of the enamel surfaces of the teeth, it is usually possible to find some surfaces of the abutment teeth that are parallel to each other. Even three widely spaced parallel lines on the teeth will be effective if they are enclosed by the framework.

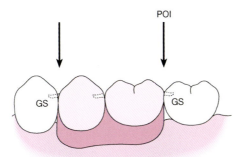

Fig 6-9 Guide surfaces (GS) parallel to the intended path of insertion restrict the possible paths of withdrawal of the partial denture.

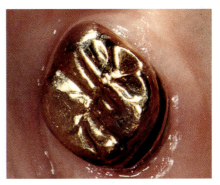

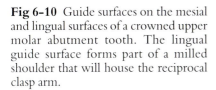

Fig 6-10 Guide surfaces on the mesial and lingual surfaces of a crowned upper molar abutment tooth. The lingual guide surface forms part of a milled shoulder that will house the reciprocal clasp arm.

Long parallel surfaces on the fitting surface of the framework can effectively act as guide surfaces. Although the tooth surfaces are not quite parallel and the denture contacts the teeth only at the surface line, such an approach can improve the stability of the path of insertion.

It is often reported that effective guide surfaces greatly reduce the reliance on clasps for retention of the partial denture. However, evidence supporting the advantages they may offer for the long-term function of partial dentures is lacking, in particular when viewed in the context of the potential long-term harm associated with partial denture use. Current concepts of partial denture design place much less emphasis on the significance of and the need for guiding surfaces and would certainly deprecate the crowning of otherwise sound abutment teeth for the sole purpose of creating effective guide surfaces.

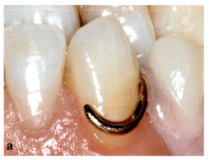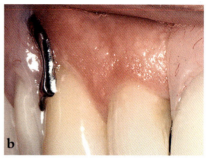

Fig 6-11 Aesthetic positioning of (a) occlusally and (b) gingivally approaching clasps.

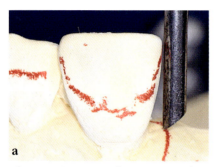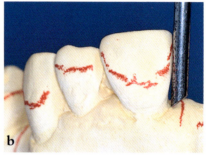

Fig 6-12 (a) Potential spacing mesial to ULI associated with the path of natural spacing. (b) The use of a path of insertion from before backwards and, in this case, a slight lateral tilt has reduced this space and will also allow the use of a labial flange.

Aesthetics

The visible display of metal components of a partial denture should be kept to a minimum. Although it may be unwise to sacrifice denture stability, poor patient acceptance can be associated with visible or unsightly clasps. Clasp tips on anterior teeth should be positioned towards the gingival margins or on the distal surfaces of the teeth (Fig 6-11). With an occlusally approaching clasp, use of a mesial undercut will allow the proximal two-thirds of the arm to remain distal to the tooth and the tip towards the gingival margin. For a gingivally approaching clasp, it may be better to use a distally placed undercut so that the arm of the retainer is less visible.

When replacing lost anterior teeth, the elimination of unsightly gaps between replacement and abutment teeth and the use of a labial flange (if required) will severely restrict the choice of a path of insertion (Fig 6-12). This will normally be from the back of the cast tilted down.

Dead spaces and interferences

Dead spaces

Any unwanted undercut area beneath the survey line on the surface of the abutment tooth next to the partial denture framework, or on other teeth enclosed by the framework, is termed "dead space" (Fig 6-13a). These represent sites where food debris can collect and stagnate and should be either minimised or kept large enough to aid natural cleansing. Dead spaces may be managed in several ways:

- The elimination of dead spaces by the removal of tooth substance (see Fig 6-9). This can be achieved by the preparation of guide surfaces and can often be performed without penetration of enamel. However, if the abutment teeth are heavily tilted, the amount of tooth tissue to be removed will be such that elimination of the dead space can only be achieved with coronal coverage restorations.
- By the deliberate enlargement of dead spaces during construction of the partial denture (Fig 6-13b). This results in "hygienic" open saddle–abutment relationship and commonly applies to posterior tooth-supported saddles. In this case, retention relative to the path of natural displacement must be provided by clasp arms that engage undercut relative to this displacement.
- By choosing a path of insertion that eliminates the unwanted undercut areas (Fig 6-13c). This approach has the additional advantage of avoiding unsightly gaps between the abutment and replacement teeth in particular, when replacing anterior teeth. It further offers the functional advantage of resisting displacement by allowing placement of rigid parts of the denture in areas undercut relative to the path of displacement. The presence of posterior bounded saddle, frequently results in an increase in dead space mesial to the distal abutment tooth.

Although food accumulation can inconvenience the patient, the effect of either the elimination of dead spaces (a closed saddle–abutment relationship) or their enlargement (an open saddle–abutment relationship) is not proved. Although there are functional and aesthetic advantages associated with the reduction of dead spaces, the concern to eliminate dead spaces *per se* is not justified and the establishment of effective plaque removal is of much greater significance for the long-term effectiveness of a partial denture.

Interferences

Teeth and soft tissues may be formed or positioned so as to physically obstruct

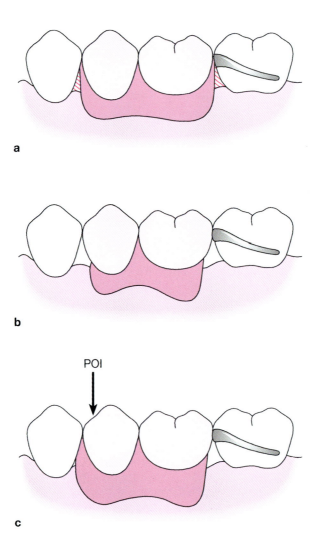

Fig 6-13 Dead spaces between the saddle and abutment teeth (a) managed by deliberate enlargement (b) and a path of insertion (POI) that eliminates the unwanted dead space distal to the mesial abutment tooth (c).

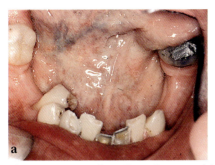 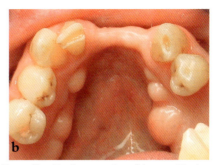

Fig 6-14 Examples of interferences: (a) lingually tilted premolar; (b) mandibular tori.

the placement of rigid denture components along an otherwise appropriate path of insertion (Fig 6-14). They are then said to act as interferences. Perhaps the most common are lingually tilted premolars and incisors. Other examples are mandibular tori that prevent the use of lingual major connectors, and bony enlargements of the edentulous ridge that prevent the normal extension of the denture saddle.

A path of insertion that avoids interferences may result in a poor distribution of retentive undercuts and a compromised appearance. In such instances, consideration should be given to the removal of interferences to allow a more appropriate path of insertion and will result in a more functional prosthesis.

Practical Surveying

It is the dentist's responsibility to design a partial denture that is both effective and relevant to the patient's dental status. Surveying is an essential part of the design process that identifies an appropriate path of insertion, allowing partial denture designs that provide effective retention and minimise the aesthetic limitations. Regrettably, several surveys have shown that the majority of practitioners abrogate this responsibility to the dental technician, a practice justified by reasons such as a lack of time, confidence or skills. It is the present author's strong contention that the design of partial dentures, including surveying, is a clinician's responsibility. A technician will simply not have the clinical information necessary to establish a partial denture design that is appropriate to the individual patient. To facilitate this clinical responsibility, a simple and logical system for effective and relevant designs for partial dentures that can be easily followed by a practitioner is described in Chapter 9 (Clinical Guide II: Establishing the Denture Design).

Key Points

- Cast surveying is an essential element of the design process for partial dentures that establishes an appropriate path of insertion.
- The path of insertion is determined by a consideration of retention and aesthetics and, to a lesser extent, guide surfaces, dead spaces and interferences.
- Once the path of insertion has been chosen, the design of the denture can be completed.
- Designing partial dentures is a clinician's responsibility and should not be delegated to the dental technician.

Chapter 7
Transitional Partial Dentures

Aim

This chapter describes partial dentures used as interim prostheses to maintain patients' appearance and function during the period of provision of definitive restorative treatment or as an aid to the transition to edentulousness.

Outcome

After reading this chapter the practitioner should be aware of the indications for the use and the design of transitional partial dentures. It should be possible to recognise the circumstances when the use of definitive partial dentures is no longer possible and a planned transition to edentulousness is necessary, a gradual process that can be effectively aided by the use of transitional, trainer partial dentures.

Introduction

Partial dentures are often used as an interim treatment that serves to maintain appearance and to provide and maintain occlusal stability during the implementation of treatment to definitively restore a partially edentulous mouth. They are also used as an aid to the transition to edentulousness when the eventual loss of all remaining teeth and the use of complete dentures seem inevitable. These partial dentures are by nature temporary and are termed transitional partial dentures.

Design of Transitional Dentures

The principles of design already established for definitive partial dentures apply equally to transitional dentures. However, given their temporary nature, it is usual to simplify the design and construction by making the dentures in acrylic resin and by deriving support from the mucosa (Fig 7-1). A broad extension of the denture base is an important design feature that is used to both minimise the load acting on the mucosa and to ensure rigidity of the denture given the relative weakness of acrylic resin. Retention is gained

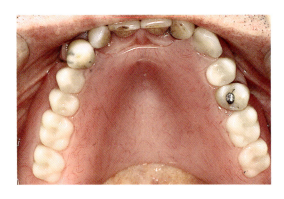

Fig 7-1 A simple all-acrylic mucosally supported transitional upper partial denture demonstrating broad extension of the denture base and tight contacts between the denture and abutment teeth.

from adhesive forces acting under the fitting surface of the broadly extended base, from tight point contacts between the replacement and abutment teeth and, in the longer term, from patient muscular control.

These simple, all-acrylic mucosally supported partial dentures have a high potential for long-term damage to the periodontal tissues and edentulous alveolar ridge. Therefore these dentures should not "progress" from the transitional to the permanent. This tendency to cause harm can be minimised in several ways:

- Clearing the denture base from the gingival margin by at least 3 mm. This is frequently possible with upper transitional dentures and is possible even if further tooth loss is anticipated as extension of the acrylic base to include further replacement teeth is technically a simple matter. Difficulties arise with lower dentures where the need for strength and rigidity of the acrylic connector will dictate a plate design. Clearance of the gingival margin can be achieved with wrought steel lingual bars although their fit and comfort are rarely satisfactory and the addition of further anterior teeth is difficult.
- The provision of tooth support with wrought or cast rests embedded within the processed acrylic. This is particularly desirable where the gingival margin is covered or where the long-term treatment plan results in prolonged use of a transitional partial denture.
- Additional retention may be gained with wrought or cast retainers. Wrought retainers are simple to fabricate but are not usually a precise fit. Cast clasps offer a more precise fit and additional tooth support through an integral occlusal rest but they do require more technical time. They may often, however, be made with other castings by attaching the wax pattern to the sprue system of another casting. Both are then

invested and cast together. This reduces considerably the time required for casting.

Examples of transitional partial dentures illustrating these features are shown in Fig 7-2.

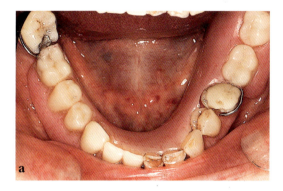

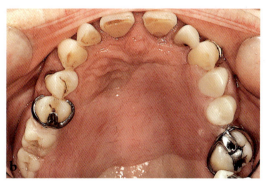

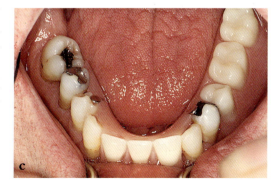

Fig 7-2 Design of transitional partial dentures. (a) Clearance of the gingival margin is rarely possible in the lower arch – simple stainless steel clasps have been used for additional retention. (b) Unnecessary gingival coverage is easily avoided in the upper arch. Cast clasps have been added for more effective support and retention. (c) Wrought stainless steel rests.

Indications for Transitional Partial Dentures

Excluding for the moment the important indication – an aid to the transition to complete denture use – common indications for the use of transitional partial dentures are as follows.

Immediate partial dentures

When the extraction of anterior teeth is required a transitional denture may be used for aesthetic reasons and as a space maintainer during the initial period of rapid bone resorption and remodelling. It is usual to complete construction of the denture before tooth extraction and fit it immediately after extractions are completed – hence the term immediate partial denture (Fig 7-3). This denture will then be replaced with a definitive partial denture or fixed prosthesis when the ridge shape has stabilised, usually three to six months after the teeth have been extracted. It is unwise to construct immediate partial dentures with cast metal frameworks as it is often not possible to try the framework in the mouth before completion with embarrassing consequences if it does not fit.

Prolonged restorative treatment

The definitive replacement for missing teeth should not be constructed until the restorative and periodontal status of the remaining teeth has been corrected and stabilised. Such treatment is frequently prolonged and partial dentures may be required for aesthetic and possibly functional reasons during provision of this treatment (Fig 7-4). In addition, periodontal treatment, particularly when it involves surgical intervention, frequently results in considerable changes to the shape of the supporting soft tissues. It is usual to

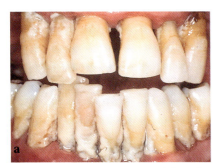 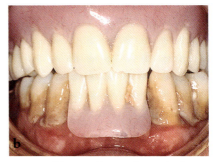

Fig 7-3 (a) Lower incisors with hopeless prognosis. (b) Use of a simple acrylic lower partial denture as their immediate replacement. All remaining upper teeth were replaced with a complete immediate denture.

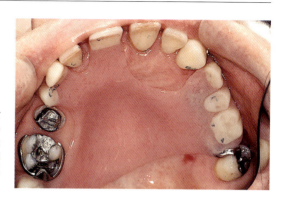

Fig 7-4 A transitional upper partial denture used to maintain appearance and occlusion during treatment to address the periodontal condition and restoration of posterior teeth.

construct transitional acrylic partial dentures that will be replaced after the periodontal treatment is successfully completed and the soft tissue shape has stabilised.

The provision of transitional partial dentures is often indicated when treating severe tooth wear and an associated loss of occlusal face height (Fig 7-5). These dentures are used to both replace missing teeth and establish a stable occlusion at an acceptable occlusal face height before and during the provision of permanent crowns, fixed and removable prosthesis. The use of transitional partial dentures to determine solely what increase in occlusal face height is acceptable to a patient is generally unnecessary since the very large majority of partially dentate patients will readily accept the increase in face height needed to restore a satisfactory appearance. When transitional partial dentures are not required to replace missing teeth, the use of simple adhesive composite restorations to effect the initial increase in face height is preferred (Fig 7-6).

Age

In young partially dentate patients it may not be feasible to provide a permanent restoration during the growing period and as a consequence a series of transitional dentures may be required. In children with hypodontia, the definitive replacement of missing teeth is frequently delayed until the eruption of permanent teeth and any necessary orthodontic tooth movement has been completed. When the planned definitive restoration of congenitally absent teeth is an implant-supported prosthesis, implant placement will not usually commence until growth has ceased. In the interim, there may be aesthetic and functional demands that can be met by the provision of transitional partial dentures. This is commonly the case for patients with

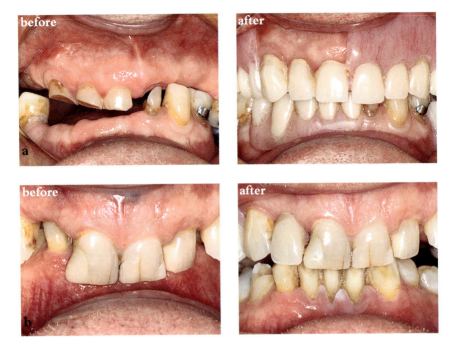

Fig 7-5 (a,b) Examples of transitional partial dentures used as an interim treatment to restore appearance and increase face height.

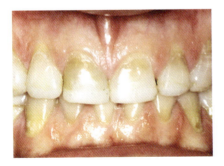

Fig 7-6 Use of simple adhesive composite restorations to restore appearance and occlusal face height without recourse to a partial denture. (Courtesy of Mr R. Tones.)

severe hypodontia in whom the use of simple mucosal borne and overlay partial dentures to replace teeth and restore occlusal face height can effect a considerable improvement in appearance and function (Fig 7-7). Such prosthesis may also act as space maintainers following completion of active orthodontic treatment. When further growth and tooth eruption is antic-

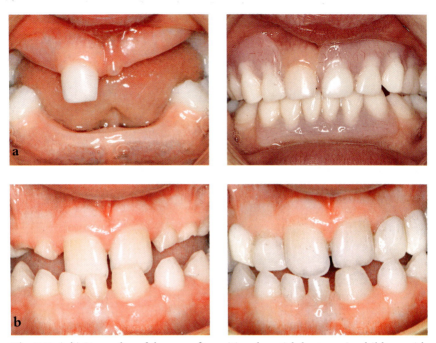

Fig 7-7 (a,b) Examples of the use of transitional partial dentures in children with severe hypodontia.

ipated, the denture will normally be all-acrylic to allow for easy adjustment and replacement, although denture fracture and loss is a potential disadvantage. In the majority of cases, sufficient improvement in both appearance and function can be made through the provision of an upper denture only. This facilitates the use of a design that will avoid unnecessary tissue damage and improve acceptance.

Examples of Commonly Used Transitional Dentures

Spoon denture

This is a useful temporary expedient when an anterior tooth is lost (Fig 7-8). The spoon denture relies on the forces of adhesion and cohesion for retention and requires a labial flange to prevent displacement palatally and rotation under occlusal loading. This design has the advantage of not covering the gingiva but it is not very stable or retentive and is of aesthetic value only.

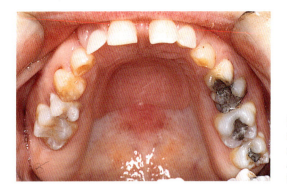

Fig 7-8 A spoon denture replacing UR2. Additional retention can be gained with Adam's cribs on posterior teeth.

Transitional partial denture with metal rests and clasps

The additional support and retention gained by the use or wrought or cast rests and clasps is desirable when prolonged use of the denture is anticipated (see Fig 7-2b). Indeed, cast clasp assemblies confer many of the functional benefits associated with cast alloy frameworks. Such a design is particularly useful in the upper arch where a prolonged period of use is envisaged. This is frequently the case following extensive periodontal treatment. Should future extractions be required, replacement teeth can be simply added to the acrylic major connector.

The Every denture

This is a simple, all-acrylic upper partial denture that may be used for bounded saddles with anterior modification spaces (Fig 7-9). It is not applicable to free-end saddles or lower partial dentures. The design was originally proposed by Every in 1949 in an attempt to overcome what was considered to be potentially destructive effects of, in particular, lateral loads on the remaining teeth. Design features of importance include:

- point contact between adjacent standing and artificial teeth
- clearance of the gingival margin palatally and an open saddle–abutment relationship
- labial and buccal flanges to assist bracing
- contact of the denture with the distal surface of the most posterior tooth to prevent distal drift and maintain the mesiodistal width of the saddle. This contact is normally achieved using stainless steel wire and has the additional benefit of augmenting retention as the labial flange and the distal surface of the last molar are often undercut with respect to each other.

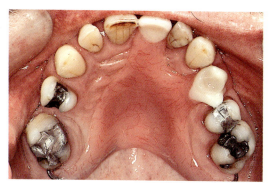

Fig 7-9 The Every denture demonstrating clearance of the gingival margin, open saddle–abutment relationship and stainless steel arms making point contact on the distal surfaces of the last standing molar teeth.

Clearance of the gingival margin makes this design useful, in particular, for those patients undergoing extensive periodontal therapy but who require replacement of missing anterior teeth.

The Transition to Edentulousness

The dental practitioner is sometimes faced with the problems of formulating treatment plans for patients who have allowed dental disease to progress to such advanced stages that multiple extractions are indicated. In some of these cases, it may become impossible or impractical to retain natural teeth to provide long-term support of partial dentures. Such patients will ultimately become edentulous and must face the prospect of wearing complete dentures. Complete dentures are not an adequate substitute for natural teeth and there are, in particular, aesthetic and functional limitations associated with their long-term use. The decision to render a patient edentulous is therefore one of last resort and must be based upon a careful evaluation of the mouth and the patient's expectations. This assessment should identify teeth that may usefully serve as overdenture abutments when the transition to complete dentures is made (Fig 7-10). This may often be the case for canine teeth and is of particular importance in the lower arch where the use of complete overdentures offers important functional advantages over conventional complete dentures. Indeed, treatment aimed to retain such teeth as potential overdenture abutments should form an essential part of the overall treatment strategy to facilitate the transition to complete denture use.

Further examples of clinical situations where a planned transition to edentulousness may be indicated are illustrated in Fig 7-11. In many cases, the number and status of the remaining teeth make the decision clear cut but

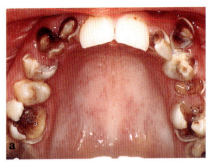 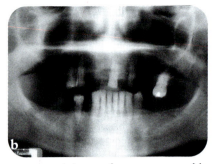

Fig 7-10 (a) Extensive caries suggests that most remaining teeth are not restorable and require extraction. Too few teeth will remain to support a definitive partial denture and the use of a transitional partial denture to ease the transition to the eventual loss of all teeth is indicated. (b) Although the prognosis for the majority or remaining upper teeth is hopeless, UR3 and UL3 could be potential overdenture abutments that will greatly improve the function of an upper complete denture.

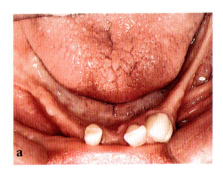 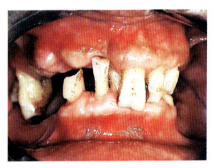

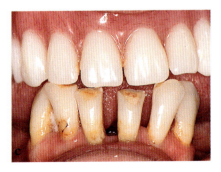

Fig 7-11 Planning for the eventual loss of all teeth. (a) The number and status of remaining teeth will not support a definitive partial denture. (b) The combination of overeruption, alveolar down growth and some over closure prevents the construction of functional definitive partial dentures. The severely overerupted teeth will require extraction and a lower complete overdenture using LR3 and LL3 as abutments and a transitional upper partial denture may be the best option. (c) Although retention of the remaining lower teeth is possible, the arch is opposed by a complete upper denture that is inherently unstable because of the poor support potential of the residual upper edentulous ridge. In this case, a complete lower overdenture may be a more functional option than a partial denture.

this is not always the case and the distribution of the remaining teeth and the status of the opposing arch can be important factors. The general health of the patient can be a further influence. For example, the likelihood of deterioration in a patient's health may dictate the early extraction of teeth of dubious prognosis as later extractions may prove hazardous. The removal of teeth of poor prognosis before radiation therapy (for malignancy) may be indicated where the mouth is within the target field.

Trainer partial dentures

Formerly, the transition to edentulousness tended to be an abrupt process typically involving the extraction of numerous teeth and the provision of complete immediate dentures. More recently, this process of total tooth loss has radically altered with a move away from the removal of large numbers of teeth to one of the gradual loss of teeth and a more gentle transition to edentulousness. This process of transition is normally effected by simple, acrylic mucosal borne transitional partial dentures that are specifically designed for later conversion into complete dentures. An important objective of providing such dentures is to give the patient an opportunity to develop denture wearing skills before all the remaining teeth are lost – hence, the term "trainer dentures".

The exact procedure will depend upon individual circumstances but often the first stage involves extraction of all or most of the posterior teeth that need to be removed. After a period of up to several months, when the posterior alveolar ridges have reached a relatively stable condition, the transitional dentures are constructed. After wearing these dentures for a limited period they may then be converted in one stage into complete dentures (Fig 7-12). More usually, successive additions of teeth are made to the dentures until the dental clearance is complete with teeth extracted as and when the need arises. This approach is generally less traumatic for patients many of whom can derive significant function from seemingly hopeless teeth for surprisingly long periods of time, delaying the eventual use of complete dentures.

To make immediate additions of artificial teeth to a denture, an impression is made of the mouth with the denture *in situ*. The denture is left in the impression during pouring of the cast, and following removal of the impression from the cast, the teeth to be replaced are cut away one by one. Each tooth removed is replaced by an artificial tooth that occupies the same position. After trimming the gingival regions to accommodate any immediate soft tissue collapse after extraction, the artificial teeth are fixed to the den-

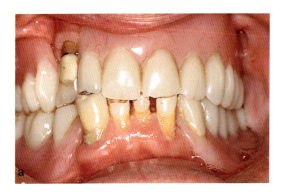

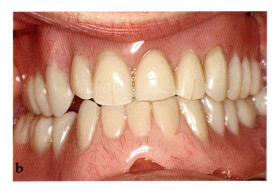

Fig 7-12 Conversion of (a) simple transitional partial dentures to (b) complete dentures.

ture with self-curing acrylic resin and the flange is completed. Finally the extractions are carried out and the converted dentures are inserted at the same appointment. The advantages and disadvantages of this use of transitional partial dentures to aid the transition to complete dentures are described in Table 7-1.

When suitable overdenture abutment teeth have been identified, the addition of the overlying replacement denture teeth will be made as a part of the final conversion to complete dentures. Necessary endodontic treatment is usually performed prior to the addition of the artificial tooth to the partial denture at which time the tooth is decoronated and prepared as an overdenture abutment (Fig 7-13).

If satisfactory partial dentures are already worn by the patient then it may be possible to convert these into complete dentures by the process of immediate

Table 7-1 **Advantages and disadvantages of the use of transitional partial dentures to aid the transition to edentulousness**

Advantages	Disadvantages
Simple and economic.	Repeated additions to denture may be socially inconvenient.
Relatively atraumatic.	Problems from remaining teeth at any time.
Function and appearance maintained.	Difficulty constructing a functional and aesthetic denture.
Can use information given by remaining teeth (e.g. vertical dimension).	Position and distribution of remaining teeth unacceptable.
Patient preference.	Prolonged treatment.
Adaptation to dentures.	

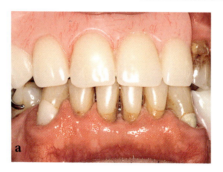

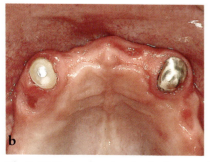
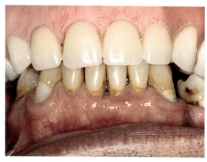

Fig 7-13 Series showing the final conversion of a transitional partial denture to a complete overdenture: (a) transitional denture in place prior to an impression of the denture *in situ* and the addition of UL3 and UL4 to the denture; (b) UL4 has been extracted and UL3 prepared as an overdenture abutment; (c) the immediate insertion of the modified denture.

additions. However, existing partial dentures are rarely adequate for this purpose but they may be used as interim prosthesis for the addition of any remaining posterior teeth, until conventional complete immediate replacement dentures are constructed.

Key Points

- Transitional partial dentures serve an important role as an interim means of restoring and maintaining appearance and occlusal stability.
- Indications include their use as immediate replacement partial dentures, as interim prosthesis during prolonged restorative treatment and in young patients in whom further growth and tooth eruption will occur.
- Simple trainer partial dentures have a significant role in the gradual transition to edentulousness.

Chapter 8
Clinical Guide I: Gathering the Information

Aim

This chapter considers the process of assessment and treatment planning for partially dentate patients. The clinical stages used to produce articulated study casts are described and the advantages of a diagnostic anterior set-up when anterior teeth are to be replaced are explained.

Outcome

After reading this chapter, the practitioner should be aware of the need for a thorough process of assessment and evaluation before embarking on treatment to replace teeth in partially dentate patients. The practitioner should be aware of the clinical procedures to produce articulated study casts and appreciate the need for an anterior try-in before the denture framework is made.

Introduction

This and the subsequent chapters outline the clinical stages involved in the provision of partial dentures and is written from the perspective that a partial denture with a metal framework is the likely treatment option for the restoration of a partially dentate patient. Each stage is described in terms of its clinical objectives and the techniques and materials required together with a discussion of the most common clinical errors. Completion of a single stage may require more than one clinical appointment.

Examination and Preliminary Impressions

The objectives of this stage are to:
• complete an initial evaluation
• make preliminary (study cast) impressions
• select an appropriate shade and mould when replacing missing anterior teeth
• carry out or arrange any necessary investigations (e.g. additional radiographs and vitality tests of potential abutment teeth).

Initial evaluation

The aims of the initial evaluation are: to diagnose any existing pathology; to identify changes that have occurred as a result of tooth loss (such changes would include poor appearance, impaired masticatory function and loss of occlusal stability); and to assess the adequacy of any existing prosthesis. The basis of this initial evaluation will be a careful and thorough case history and examination. Whilst this approach does not differ in any particular way from that for the fully dentate patient, there are certain aspects which are of relevance to partially dentate patients. For convenience these are considered under the headings of case history and examination.

Case history

Complaints relating to poor appearance and loss of masticatory function are frequently made by partially dentate patients. The exact nature and extent of such complaints must be clearly established by further questioning. The past history of tooth loss and any prosthesis constructed subsequent to tooth loss must be identified. The usual causes of tooth loss are caries, periodontal disease and trauma. The patient's evaluation of any existing prosthesis must be sought and the reasons for any dissatisfaction determined.

Examination

The examination must establish the periodontal, caries and pulpal status of the remaining natural teeth, the adequacy of existing restorations and identify existing soft tissue pathology. With regard to possible future provision of prosthesis, particular note should be made of the following:

- The edentulous ridges – Features such as the amount of resorption, the health and consistency of the supporting soft tissue, prominent fraenal attachments and the presence of bony exostoses and unfavourable bony undercuts should be noted (Fig 8-1).
- Loss of occlusal stability – This can be assessed by the identification of tilting, rotation, drifting and overeruption of teeth, and the examination of the number and pattern of tooth contacts in intercuspal position (ICP), retruded, lateral and protrusive occlusion (Fig 8-2).
- The space available for a prosthesis – Examples include the overeruption of unopposed teeth; a deep, complete overbite in relation to missing anterior teeth and commonly seen in Class II malocclusions; and the reduced interdental space that often results from tooth wear (Fig 8-3).
- The existing partial denture(s) – This should be carefully assessed both in and out of the mouth with regard to appearance, fit, retention and stability, and the adequacy of its design and the possible harm it may be causing to the remaining teeth and supporting soft tissues (Fig 8-4).

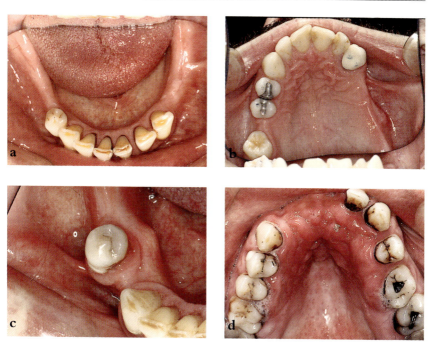

Fig 8-1 Examination of the edentulous ridges. (a) Well formed and firm lower edentulous ridges. (b) Moderate to severe resorption of the edentulous ridge – note the presence of the prominent buccal fraenum. (c) Lingual bony exostoses and prominent buccal fraenum in relationship to the single standing premolar. (d) Denture-induced stomatitis with reddening and slight papillomatous changes confined to the region of palatal coverage by an upper partial denture.

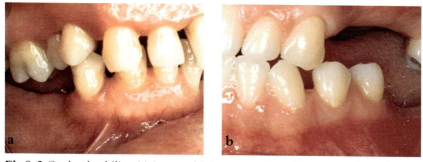

Fig 8-2 Occlusal stability. (a) An unstable intercuspation with overeruption of unopposed posterior teeth and spacing and drifting of anterior teeth related to loss of lower posterior teeth and periodontal involvement. (b) A stable occlusion with only slight evidence of tooth movement despite the loss of posterior teeth.

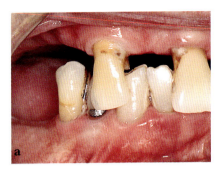
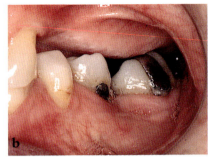
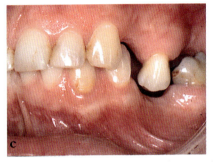
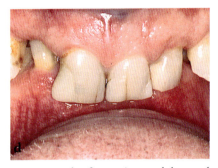

Fig 8-3 Space for prosthesis. (a,b) Overclosure as a result of posterior tooth loss and anterior tooth wear, and some overeruption of LR5 in (a) has severely limited the space available for a prosthesis. (c) Overeruption of the unopposed UL5 together with alveolar bone down growth. There is no evidence of significant overclosure. (d) The loss of stable posterior contacts in a Class II division 2 malocclusion has accentuated the severe overbite and eliminated any space for a prosthesis.

In the light of this initial diagnosis and evaluation, it may be necessary to plan for some preliminary treatment to provide immediate relief of symptoms and the stabilisation of progressive disease. The initiation of primary preventive measures (e.g. oral hygiene instruction and fluoride application) and secondary prevention (e.g. initiation of non-surgical management of periodontal disease and the removal of other plaque retentive factors such as deficient restorations) may often be required at this early stage. This initial treatment may also involve adjustment of an existing partial denture that may be damaging teeth or soft tissues or require the immediate addition of one or more teeth.

Articulated study casts
Articulated study casts are an essential adjunct to the evaluation and treat-

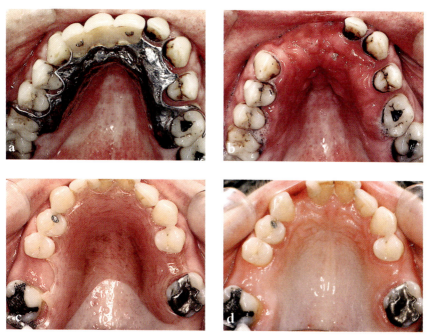

Fig 8-4 Existing dentures. (a,b) An ill-fitting and poorly designed cobalt-chromium partial denture associated with denture-induced stomatitis and palatal decalcification of several teeth. Such effects are not inevitable. The poorly fitting acrylic upper partial denture with extensive gingival coverage shown in (c) has not been associated with a deterioration of the health of the hard and soft tissues (d).

ment planning for a partially dentate patient and have the following uses:
- Indication of loss of hard and soft tissues.
- Surveying and design of partial dentures.
- Occlusal analysis.
- Indicate necessary tooth preparations.
- Anterior set-ups and diagnostic wax-ups for assessment at the chairside.

Preliminary (study cast) impressions

The preparation of useful preliminary impressions of partially dentate patients can be challenging since it combines the requirements for an accurate and detailed record of any remaining teeth together with the need to capture the full extent and detail of the potential denture-bearing area. Alginate is the impression material of choice but, unless this can be supported by well-extended and rigid stock dentate impression trays, modification of the impression tray to achieve an adequate extension and support of the alginate impression material will be required. Thermoplastic impression compound is a useful material in this regard and its addition may often be necessary in the vault of the palate, over large edentulous areas (three or more missing teeth) and in lingual and buccal sulci if the tray flange appears short in these areas (Fig 8-5). Any impression compound that flows close to the teeth should be trimmed back to allow a minimum of 3 mm space for the alginate. A detailed impression of the teeth can be ensured by simply drying the teeth with gauze and then wiping a small quantity of alginate into the occlusal fissures and embrasure immediately before seating the loaded impression tray.

Further investigations
Additional investigations will usually be required. These should include up-to-date radiographs of all potential abutment teeth and any other tooth considered to have doubtful prognosis. The most useful radiograph is a dental panoramic tomograph (DPT) but this should be augmented with intraoral views in areas that are not sufficiently detailed by the DPT (Fig 8-6). It is normally wise to perform vitality tests of carious and restored abutment teeth, together with other carious or heavily restored teeth that may be involved in the design of a prosthesis.

Further opinions with respect to diagnosis or, more frequently, treatment planning may form a part of this continuing evaluation. Common examples of such opinions may include the prognosis of periodontally involved teeth, and the possibility and design of fixed or removable prosthesis. It is important that as much information as possible is made available to inform the treatment planning.

Common errors
- Insufficient attention paid to the existing occlusion.
- Incomplete impression of the palate due to insufficient material or, much more commonly, a failure to seat the tray completely often as a result of overloading the impression material.
- Poor recording of the lingual sulcus due either to inadequate modification of the tray or because the tongue was not elevated and forward when taking the impression.
- Deficiency in the labial sulcus. The mouth was open too wide when the tray was being seated. The lip was not relaxed and lifted forward to allow impression material to flow into the sulcus.

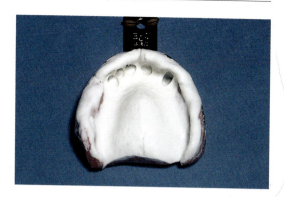

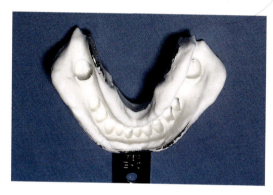

Fig 8-5 Upper and lower preliminary (study cast) impressions that have recorded the detail of the remaining teeth and the full extent of the potential denture-bearing areas. In the upper, this has required the use of impression compound to support alginate in the large edentulous areas and the palate.

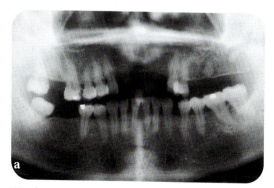

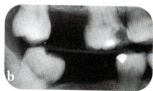

Fig 8-6 Radiographic examination. (a) In many cases, a dental panoramic tomograph alone will provide sufficient detail of the mouth as a whole but should be supplemented by intraoral views (b) as is necessary.

97

Preliminary Registration and Denture Design

The objectives of this stage are to:
- complete a preliminary jaw registration (if required)
- try in anterior teeth where relevant, and modify as necessary.

Preliminary registration

A preliminary registration may be necessary to allow articulation of the study casts. The nature of this registration will vary (Fig 8-7). For most partially dentate patients, the jaw relationship record is made in the existing intercuspal position. The essential requirement of this registration is that it should facilitate accurate articulation of the study casts by providing a stable record of the intercuspal position. This is achieved by ensuring bilateral contact(s) in the posterior and anterior regions. Where there are few missing teeth it may be possible simply to "hand articulate" the casts. More usually, wax occlusal rims and an additional registration stage is necessary. It should, however, be emphasised that these simply provide the means of obtaining a stable record of the intercuspal position, the orientation of the occlusal plane and the occlusal face height will be dictated by the natural teeth.

Where an existing intercuspal position is considered to be unsuitable and/or when further occlusal assessment is required, then the retruded contact position is used as the mandibular reference position for mounting study casts. In such circumstances study casts should be mounted on a semi-adjustable articulator. This requires the use of a pre-contact registration on the retruded arc of closure of the mandible (a retruded axis record) and a facebow record. Determination of freeway space is not normally required.

An assessment of freeway space is relevant where, for reasons of tooth wear or the lack of occlusal stops, it is felt that the occlusal face height should be increased. This, together with the jaw relation record and a semi-adjustable articulator as described above will allow the accurate appraisal of various increases in occlusal face height with the articulated study casts. Although the determination of freeway space and occlusal face height is obviously relevant when one arch is edentulous, this is usually left until the definitive jaw relation record is made, a preliminary registration rarely being required.

Anterior try-in

When anterior teeth are to be replaced it is often useful to carry out an anterior try-in at an early stage in treatment. This can be combined with the preliminary registration. The advantages of an anterior try-in are particularly

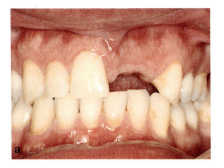
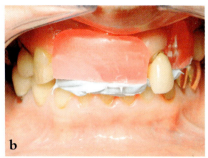

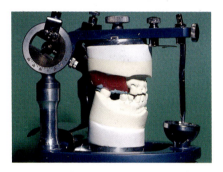

Fig 8-7 Preliminary registration. (a) Positive bilateral posterior and anterior tooth contacts will allow articulation of study casts in the intercuspal position without the need for a registration record. (b) With more extensive tooth loss an occlusal rim ensures a stable record of the existing intercuspal position. (c) Extensive posterior tooth loss and anterior tooth wear. A facebow and retruded axis record to mount study casts will allow evaluation of the change in occlusal face height needed to restore appearance.

evident, when the patient has specific aesthetic concerns or demands (Fig 8-8). An anterior set-up will:

- attend to the patient's aesthetic concerns early in treatment
- highlight the aesthetic possibilities and limitations
- allow the technician to construct a metal framework that matches the position of the replacement teeth.

As described in Chapter 4, a metal base that closely fits the supporting soft tissues of an anterior saddle leaves more space for the replacement teeth and this in turn results in a better appearance of anterior denture teeth. In addition, metal backing of the replacement anterior teeth improves the long-term retention of the anterior denture teeth when interocclusal space is limited. A silicone or plaster matrix of the arrangement of the replacement anterior teeth confirmed with an anterior try-in allows the technician to position accurately the studs or tags needed to retain the replacement teeth to the metal framework and to incorporate correctly any necessary metal backing.

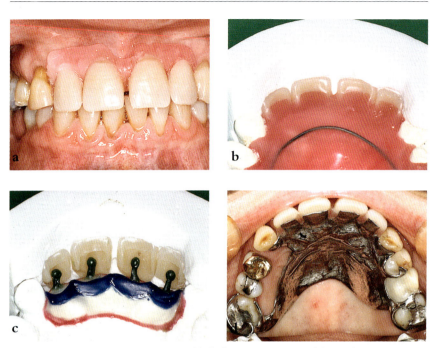

Fig 8-8 (a) An anterior try-in to establish the arrangement of the replacement anterior teeth. This is transferred to the casts on which the framework is constructed using an index of this set-up (b) and this allows accurate positioning of retention tags (c) and metal backing of the anterior denture teeth (d).

Common errors

- Teeth are apart when the casts are seated into the registration. The wax rim(s) was displaced into the supporting soft tissues because of heavy contact between natural teeth and occlusal rim or the patient closed together too firmly (never ask the patient to "bite together").
- Contact between the heels of the study casts.
- Excessive recording material was used. Its flow into occlusal fissures and embrasure spaces will often prevent accurate seating of the casts into the registration. Record opposing cusp tips only. It is always good practice to seat the jaw registration record on the study casts and to check its accuracy before the patient is dismissed.
- Insufficient attention paid to occlusion.

Definitive Treatment Plan

The objectives of this stage are to discuss and confirm the treatment plan with the patient. It is at this stage that a decision about the definitive treatment is normally made. The principal objectives when treating partially dentate patients are to preserve the remaining teeth in a stable and healthy environment, to prevent further pathological change and, if necessary, to restore function. The collation of information obtained should enable the clinician to determine the following:

- Treatment necessary to restore and maintain the remaining dentition in health.
- The need to replace missing teeth and, where this need exists, the treatment involved in the alternative means of replacing them. With regards to the possible use of a partial denture, this decision may have to await the surveying and design procedure (see Chapter 9).
- The treatment most appropriate for the patient. Factors of importance will be the patient's expectations of treatment, their ability to attain and maintain adequate plaque control, their ability to attend for regular treatment and later maintenance, possible complications arising from the patient's medical history and, by no means least, economic considerations. It should be remembered that many partially dentate patients are elderly and in the short or long-term may present dental management difficulties resulting from a deteriorating oral hygiene, poor health and poly pharmacy and a worsening, often cariogenic, diet.

Key Points

- Treatment of partially dentate patients should be based upon an assessment of the patient's complaints and demands and a thorough clinical examination.
- In addition to establishing the dental status of remaining teeth, the examination should include an assessment of the potential denture-bearing areas, occlusal relationships and the availability of space for a prosthesis.
- Articulated study casts are an essential aid to the treatment planning process.
- The patient's general health, medical and social history can have a profound influence on the choice of treatment.

Chapter 9
Clinical Guide II: Establishing the Denture Design

Aim

This chapter will present a simple and logical system, which when followed, will produce effective and relevant designs for partial dentures.

Outcome

After reading this chapter, the practitioner should be able to apply the recommended, simple and logical system of partial denture design.

Introduction

The dental surveyor and the broad principles underlying the use of cast surveying to establish the design of a partial denture were described in Chapter 6. Using a simple design sheet, a surveyor and study cast(s), follow the procedure set out below. For convenience, the study cast(s) should be "split-cast" mounted on the articulator to allow them to be separated from the mounting plaster and securely placed on the cast table (Fig 9-1). Comment and suggestions are given for each step in the design process.

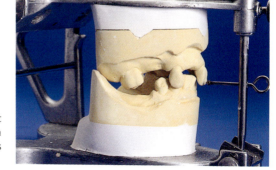

Fig 9-1 Study casts split-cast mounted to allow separation of the upper cast from its mounting plaster.

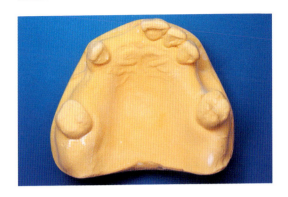

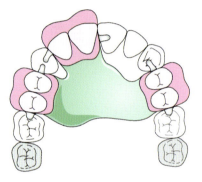

Fig 9-2 Step 1: There is no functional need to replace the missing last molars. Rests have been added at each end of the saddles and a simple major connector to join the saddles outlined. (Colour coding can help to clarify the design – in this case: green for cobalt-chromium and pink for acrylic.)

Step 1

Decide which teeth are to be replaced and outline the saddle areas. Provide tooth support for the saddles with rests. Outline a simple major connector (Fig 9-2).

Comments
- Not all missing teeth need to be replaced.
- Although a ranking order of useful support would run from first molars down to lower incisors, pragmatically one simply uses the abutment teeth available. Even teeth with marked loss of attachment can provide useful tooth support.
- The design of the major connector is normally decided when the denture design is finalised and, in the lower arch, may sometimes be delayed until the working impression has been recorded.

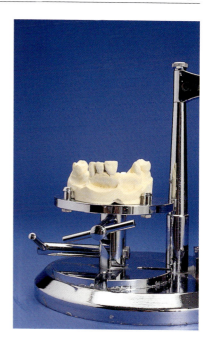

Fig 9-3 Step 2: The cast positioned on the cast table with its occlusal plane horizontal.

Suggestion
Place rests at both ends of a bounded saddle. For lower free-end saddles, mesial placement of the rest is preferred.

Step 2

Position the cast on the surveyor table with the occlusal plane approximating the horizontal (Fig 9-3).

Comment
For any one denture displacement away from the tissues may be possible in several directions. However, it is generally assumed that all partial dentures will have a tendency to withdraw along a path at right angles to the occlusal plane – the path of natural displacement (see Chapter 6).

Suggestion
Remember, undercut relative to this horizontal survey must be engaged to ensure effective retention. This can be by clasps alone or, by modifying the path of insertion, a rigid part of the denture, or a combination of both.

Step 3

Identify usable (retentive) undercut by surveying the cast with a red lead (Fig 9-4).

Comments

This undercut can normally be found on buccal, lingual and proximal surfaces of abutment teeth. It may also be present in relation to edentulous areas – for example, labial undercut in relation to an anterior edentulous space.

Retentive undercut cannot be "created" by tilting the cast. Although clasps can be designed to engage the "created" undercut, they will not prevent natural displacement as the undercut is not present relative to natural displacement.

Suggestions

If there is no usable undercut with the horizontal survey, then it must be created if natural displacement is to be resisted. An example is the creation of undercut to be engaged by a clasp by the simple addition of etch–retained composite to the buccal surface of an abutment tooth.

Step 4

Consider the influence of aesthetics and interferences on the path of insertion. Continue your examination of the cast with an analysing rod and modify the cast tilt as necessary (Fig 9-5).

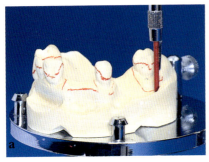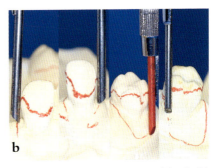

Fig 9-4 Step 3: (a) The horizontal survey has been completed using a red lead. (b) Useful retentive undercut is present on the buccal surfaces of all abutment teeth. Proximal undercut is also present on the distal surface of UL3 and, to a lesser extent, the distal surface of UR3.

Comments

When replacing lost anterior teeth, both the elimination of unsightly gaps between replacement and abutment teeth and the use of a labial flange (unless contraindicated) will often severely restrict the choice of a path of insertion. This will normally be from before backwards.

For free-end saddle dentures, it is usual to select a path of insertion that eliminates or reduces proximal undercut on the distal surface of abutment teeth if this undercut is present at the horizontal survey. This improves retention by allowing rigid parts of the saddle to resist natural displacement and is achieved by tipping the cast down at the front.

When free-end saddle dentures have anterior modification spaces, a path of insertion that ensures a good appearance will take priority over optimum retention.

Suggestions

If the path of insertion at the horizontal survey satisfies the design requirements for, in particular, retention and aesthetics, there is no need to alter it. Try to avoid paths of insertion that differ markedly from the path of natural displacement as this may cause difficulties designing clasps that resist natural displacement. For example, it is rarely necessary to extend a labial flange to the depth of the labial sulcus – this avoids the need to select a path of insertion that eliminates all labial soft tissue undercut.

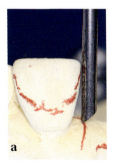 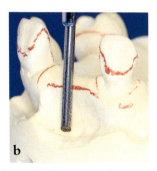 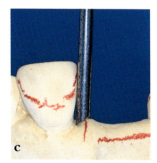

Fig 9-5 Step 4: (a) The path of insertion for the horizontal survey results in dead space mesial to UL1 and (b) deep soft tissue undercut labially that prevents the use of a labial flange. (c) A new path of insertion created by tipping the cast down at the back and slightly to the left reduces the soft tissue undercut and thus allows placement of a labial flange and minimises unsightly dead space mesial to UL1.

Step 5

When you have decided on a suitable path of insertion, lock the cast table. Using a black marking lead, map out all undercut areas on both hard and soft tissues. Mark the path of insertion on three sides of the base of the cast. Make three transfer tripod marks by marking three widely separated points on the cast that are touched by the analysing rod as it moves through a fixed horizontal plane (Fig 9-6).

Comment
Contrasting colours for the horizontal and final survey allow the ready identification of undercut common to both paths of insertion. Transfer tripod points allow the transfer of the chosen path of insertion from the study cast to the working cast.

Step 6

Complete the design of any clasps. Ensure that they are reciprocated (Fig 9-7).

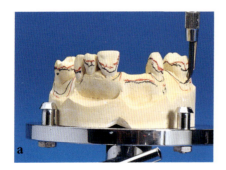
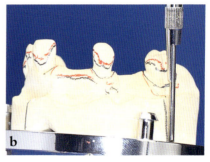
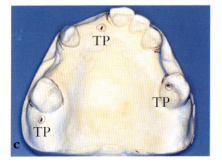

Fig 9-6 Step 5: (a) The path of insertion has been decided. The cast table is locked and the cast resurveyed using a black lead to contrast with the red of the horizontal survey. Note the change in undercut distribution. (b) The path of insertion is recorded using base markings on the study cast and (c) transfer tripod points (TP).

Comment

For most partial dentures, two effective clasps will provide sufficient retention. Ideally these should engage undercut common to both the horizontal survey and the selected path of insertion.

Suggestions

Where possible, position two clasps on a diagonal across the arch. For cobalt-chromium clasps the tip of the retentive clasp arm should engage 0.25–0.5 mm depth of undercut, for gold clasps 0.5–0.75 mm is appropriate.

Try to minimise the display of clasp arms, in particular, towards the front of the mouth. For an occlusally approaching clasp a mesial undercut allows the proximal two-thirds of the arm to be distal to the tooth and the termination

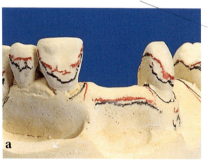
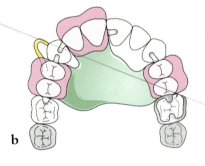

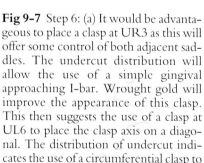

Fig 9-7 Step 6: (a) It would be advantageous to place a clasp at UR3 as this will offer some control of both adjacent saddles. The undercut distribution will allow the use of a simple gingival approaching I-bar. Wrought gold will improve the appearance of this clasp. This then suggests the use of a clasp at UL6 to place the clasp axis on a diagonal. The distribution of undercut indicates the use of a circumferential clasp to engage the mesiobuccal undercut. (b) The clasps are added to the denture design. The cingulum rest will reciprocate the retentive clasp arm at UR3. The addition of a distal rest at UL6 will ensure rigidity of the palatal part of the clasp arm which will reciprocate the terminal third entering the mesiobuccal undercut. (c) The position of the clasp tip in undercut has been marked using a 0.5 mm undercut gauge.

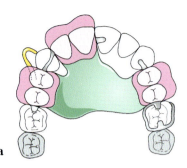
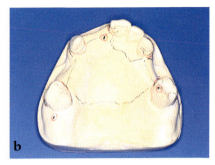

Fig 9-8 Step 7: (a) Indirect retention is not necessary and the design of the major connector is completed. Although coverage of the gingival margin is desirable, clearing the gingival margin palatally to UR3 will result in a narrow stagnation area. In this case, the connector has been extended onto UR3 and is supported by a cingulum rest. (b) It is helpful to outline the major connector on the study cast.

at the gingival margin. For a gingivally approaching clasp, it may be better to use a distal undercut so that the arm of the retainer is less visible.

If the location of undercut does not allow aesthetic placement of the clasp, consider "engineering" a more favourable undercut distribution through the simple combination of lowering survey lines and the addition of etch-retained composite (see tooth preparation in Chapter 10).

Step 7

Consider the need for indirect retention. Complete the design of the major connector (Fig 9-8).

Comments
Provision of indirect retention is only really necessary for lower free-end saddle dentures largely because components acting as indirect retainers will facilitate later reline procedures.

A connector design that leaves the gingival margins free is preferred. If the connector must cover the gingival margin, ensure adequate tooth support.

Clearance of the gingival margin is rarely a problem in the upper arch. In the lower arch there should be about 7 mm between the gingival margin and the functional depth of the lingual sulcus to ensure adequate clearance.

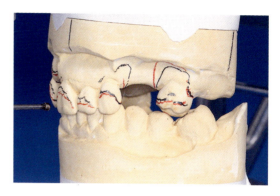

Fig 9-9 Step 8: The influence of the occlusion on the design is checked on the articulated study casts. In this case, there is room for all components. The only tooth preparations required are rest seat preparations at UR6, UR3, UL1, UL3 and UL6.

Suggestions

A simple design outweighs the theoretical advantage of indirect retention. If provision of indirect retention overcomplicates the design do not include it.

Whilst a lingual plate is the easy option if the lack of available space prevents the use of a lingual bar, consider the use of the more hygienic sublingual or dental bar.

Step 8

Finalise the design prescription (Fig 9-9).

Comment

Examine the relationship of your design to the occlusion of the natural teeth. If components of the design are likely to interfere with the occlusion, tooth preparations must be planned or the design modified.

Suggestion

Common preparations are lowering survey lines in relation to the root of clasp arms, and rest seat preparations to provide adequate clearance for rigid rests.

Common errors at this stage
- Insufficient attention paid to the occlusion.
- Failure to ensure retention along the path of natural displacement.

Key Points

- The starting point of the surveying and design procedure is the identifi-

111

cation of undercut relative to the likely path of displacement of a partial denture – the path of natural displacement.

- The introduction of denture components such as clasps or rigid parts of the partial denture to resist this displacement will ensure retention.
- The main indications for a path of insertion that differs from that of natural displacement are to improve aesthetics when anterior teeth are to be replaced and to maximise retention in free-end saddle dentures.
- Avoid the use of a path of insertion that differs markedly from the path of natural displacement.
- Interferences can profoundly influence the choice of a suitable path of insertion and may prevent the use of a partial denture.
- Clasps are designed after the path of insertion has been established.

Chapter 10

Clinical Guide III: Preparation of the Mouth for Partial Dentures

Aim

This chapter aims to describe preparations of the remaining natural teeth that are commonly required to facilitate the design of the partial denture. It will emphasise the use of simple enamel reshaping and will outline the clinical techniques used when alterations to tooth shape are incorporated into cast coronal restorations in abutment teeth.

Outcome

After reading this chapter the practitioner should be aware of the design of commonly used tooth preparations and understand how these may be achieved both by simple enamel reshaping and by incorporation into cast coronal restorations.

Introduction

There are two separate phases of mouth preparation for removable partial dentures. The first phase involves the creation of a healthy oral environment prior to construction of the prosthesis and includes periodontal, operative, endodontic, orthodontic and surgical treatment as is required. The second phase of mouth preparation involves the alteration of tooth contours to allow the proper fit and functioning of the proposed removable partial denture. It is to this phase of the mouth preparation that this chapter is devoted.

Tooth Preparation

Information gained from surveying the patient's study casts will indicate modifications of tooth structure that may be required to put the finalised denture design into practice. Modifications that are often required include:

• Preparation of guide surfaces.
• Lowering survey lines to improve clasp placement.
• Rest seat preparations.

- Creation of retentive clasp undercut.
- Embrasure widening to provide space for clasp arms passing between teeth and to allow sufficient bulk of minor connectors joining rests to the major connector.
- The reduction of interferences, e.g. proximal surfaces of teeth adjoining anterior edentulous spaces and the lingual bulge of mandibular premolars that are tipped lingually and could interfere with the placement of the framework.
- Adjustments to the level of the occlusal plane.

Tooth preparations should be planned using the articulated study casts following surveying and partial denture design. This allows a clear indication of both the position and extent of any necessary modification to the coronal contour. For most patients these preparations will be confined to abutment teeth and can be achieved by simple enamel reshaping. The routine use of crowning to achieve an ideal coronal shape is not necessary, there being little evidence that this practice confers any functional advantage. Crown preparation requires the irreversible removal of considerable amounts of tooth tissue. Crowns are subject to long-term failure and cannot be considered an adequate substitute for sound coronal tooth tissue. However, where the presence of an extensive restoration or wear indicates the need for a cast coronal restoration, this provides an ideal opportunity to incorporate any necessary rest seats, retentive undercut or guide surfaces within the restoration.

It is always good practice to list the tooth preparations required and to mark the position of these preparations on the study casts. If the preparations are then made on the study casts and the casts resurveyed to confirm that the preparations have been completed, a good estimate of the position and the extent of any preparations can be gained. Armed with this information, tooth preparation can be embarked upon with confidence.

A suggested clinical sequence for tooth preparations is as follows:
- prepare guide surfaces
- lower survey lines to allow an improved clasp location
- carry out embrasure widening
- prepare rest seats
- create retentive undercut.

It is recommended that the majority of enamel reduction is done using air rotor diamonds of the appropriate shape and size. Then further refinements are made using stones and abrasive–impregnated rubber points.

Guide surfaces

Preparation of guide surfaces requires an even and minimal reduction of enamel, following and maintaining the contour of the involved surface of the tooth. Flat preparations, using discs, are needlessly destructive of tooth tissue (Fig 10-1). Guide surfaces are most frequently prepared on the proximal surfaces of abutment teeth adjacent to the edentulous spaces. As a rule of thumb, proximal guide surfaces should be about as wide as the distance between the tips of the buccal and lingual cusps and should extend vertically 2–3 mm, or more if possible, finishing well above the gingival margin. The natural contour of a proximal surface results in the reduction of height lingually as the preparation tapers towards the lingual surface (Fig 10-2). Less commonly, guide surfaces are prepared on the lingual surface to aid clasp reciprocation. These surfaces are located on the tooth surface directly opposite the proposed site of the clasp tip.

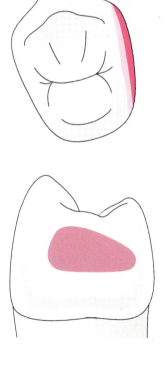

Fig 10-1 A guide surface should be prepared by even reduction of the surface of the tooth maintaining its contour (shown as red) and not as a flat surface (shown in pink).

Fig 10-2 A proximal guide surface should be 2–3 mm high and about as wide as the distance between the buccal and lingual cusps. The natural contour of the tooth results in a preparation that tapers towards the lingual surface.

115

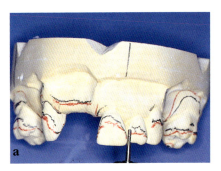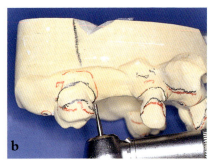

Fig 10-3 (a,b) Checking the orientation of the bur to the path of insertion on the surveyed study cast. (See marks on the base of the casts.)

During guide surface preparation the angulation of the bur required to produce a guide surface parallel to the intended path of insertion is first established on the study casts. Marking the path of insertion labially and buccally on the base of the cast will facilitate this procedure (Fig 10-3). This angulation of the bur is then transferred to the mouth by eye. Although somewhat imprecise, this simple process of "eye balling" the transfer of the path of insertion to the tooth surface can, with care, achieve reasonable parallelism for one or two guide surface preparations but is unlikely to result in sufficient accuracy for multiple preparations. Maintaining this angulation, the bur is guided around the tooth surface, all the while observing the guiding surface developing in a gingival direction, until preparation is complete (Fig 10-4). To prepare further guide surfaces the procedure is repeated.

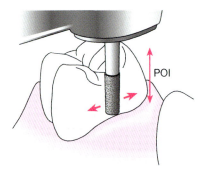

Fig 10-4 Having established the correct orientation, the cylindrical diamond bur is moved back and forth around the involved surface of the tooth. (POI, path of insertion.)

Lowering survey lines

Lowering survey lines by the reduction of tooth bulbosity is a simple and reliable technique that can improve clasp placement by allowing:

- the origin of a circumferential clasp arm to be placed well below the occlusal surface
- the retentive clasp tip to be placed in the gingival third of the crown, providing better mechanical function and aesthetics
- a reciprocal arm to be placed on and above the height of contour well below the occlusal surface.

When lowering survey lines, the initial preparation is made with the same cylindrical bur used for the preparation of the guide surfaces. Alignment is by eyeballing with reference to the intended path of insertion on the study casts. Having established the correct angulation, the bur is positioned alongside the enamel surface to be prepared. The head of the handpiece is then tipped slightly towards the long axis of the tooth. Maintaining this new angulation, enamel is removed from the involved tooth surface until the gingival part of the preparation occupies the desired position – the new, lowered survey line (Fig 10-5).

Embrasure widening

This is achieved by enlarging the lingual embrasure with a narrow tapered diamond bur (Fig 10-6). The re-contouring should blend smoothly with the lingual and proximal surfaces.

Rest seat preparation

Rest seat preparations aim to provide space for a rigid rest that does not interfere with the occlusion. In addition, the shape of the completed preparation

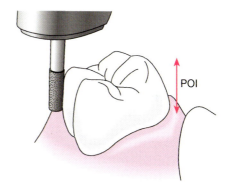

Fig 10-5 Lowering survey lines: having orientated the bur along the path of insertion (POI), the bur is placed against the involved surface, the head of the handpiece is tipped slightly towards the centre of the tooth and the survey line lowered by moving the bur back and forth.

POI

117

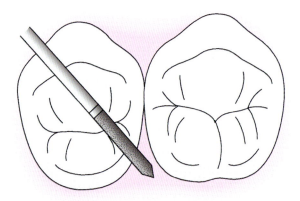

Fig 10-6 Enlarging the interproximal area.

should provide positive seating for the rest (see Occlusal rests) and should be rounded to allow some movement of the rest in function. These objectives are achieved by tooth reduction which maintains the original contour of the tooth surface.

The correct design and positioning of rest seats requires that the study casts be observed in occlusion. If possible, cingulum rests should be placed apical to the areas of contact with the opposing teeth and occlusal rest seat preparations must be sufficiently deep so that the opposing cusps do not meet the finished rest prematurely. The depth of this reduction will vary with the nature of occlusal contacts but as a general guide it should be at least 1 mm thick to ensure adequate strength of the rest. As a quick check that sufficient enamel has been removed, patients can be asked gently to close together on a strip of softened baseplate wax; the thickness of the wax in the region of the preparation will give a good indication as to whether adequate clearance has been made.

Occlusal rests
The outline of the completed occlusal rest seat preparation used for posterior teeth resembles a saucered spoon broadest at the marginal ridge and

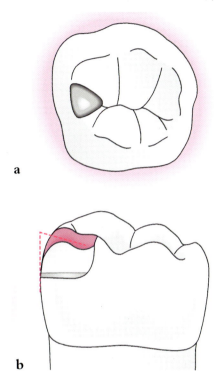

a

b

Fig 10-7 The occlusal rest seat preparation: (a) occlusal outline (b) sectional view of occlusal rest seat to show how lowering the existing contour of the tooth ensures positive seating of the rest.

tapering in towards the centre of the tooth. By maintaining but reducing the existing contour of the tooth, the deepest part of the rest will form an angle of less then 90° with the proximal surface of the tooth at the marginal ridge and will thus ensure positive seating (Fig 10-7).

The preparation is started by first reducing and rounding the middle third of the marginal ridge using a round diamond bur of an appropriate size (no. 6 for molars, no. 4 for premolars) (Fig 10-8). This is followed by deepening of the adjacent fossa which is then blended into the reduced marginal ridge. Once complete, the preparation should be examined to ensure that no interferences to the path of insertion have been created and any small enamel "lips" should be smoothed.

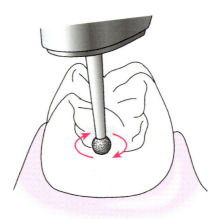

Fig 10-8 Occlusal rest seat preparation is begun by reducing and rounding the middle third of the marginal ridge.

Cingulum rests

Positive seating for a cingulum rest is created by preparing a rounded groove within enamel just above the cingulum (Fig 10-9a). This preparation is most frequently used on upper anterior teeth and, in particular, canines in which the cingulum is often sufficiently developed to allow an adequate preparation with only modest reduction of enamel. A suitable round high speed diamond bur (no. 2) is aligned with the long axis of the tooth and then angled slightly towards the centre of the tooth. A rounded groove is created by passing the rotating bur up and over and just incisal to the cingulum (Fig 10-9b). The angulation of the bur results in a groove that is deepest towards the centre of the tooth thus ensuring a positive seating for the rest. The groove should broaden proximally where the rest joins the framework to ensure adequate strength at this point. Preparation frequently results in a lip of enamel incisal to the rest seat preparation. This lip should be blended into the remaining lingual contour.

Incisal rests

The steep vertical slope and poorly developed cingulum often seen on the lingual surface of lower anterior teeth prevents the preparation of cingulum

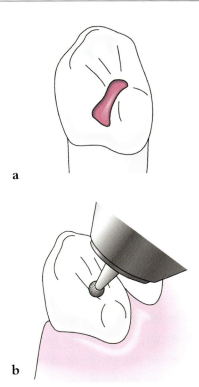

Fig 10-9 (a) Semilunar outline of prepared cingulum rest. (b) Bur positioned just incisal to the cingulum and angled towards the centre of the tooth.

rest seats without penetration of enamel. This may be overcome either by the augmentation of the cingulum by bonded composite additions or with an incisal rest. The major disadvantage of the incisal rest is a poor appearance resulting from the inevitable display of metal at the incisal edge. However, with care both in the site of the rest and the fabrication of the framework these aesthetic problems can be minimised.

Initial preparation consists of a notch cut into the incisal edge using a flame shaped diamond bur. This notch should be positioned 1–2 mm. in from the mesial or distal incisal corner and should slope towards the lingual in an attempt to keep extension on to the labial surface to a minimum. The notch should be blended into the lingual surface contour and bevelled labially (Fig 10-10).

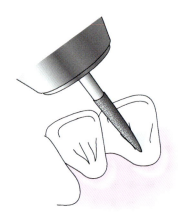

Fig 10-10 Incisal rest seat preparation: the notch is prepared 1–2 mm in from the mesial or distal incisal corner and the bur should be angled towards the lingual in an attempt to keep extension on to the labial surface to a minimum.

Creation of clasp undercut

The simplest method of creating a retentive undercut for a clasp is with an adhesive composite addition to the involved tooth surface (Fig 10-11). This assumes that there is a sufficient quantity and quality of enamel to ensure an adequate bond and that the position and morphology of the tooth allows the creation of undercut without an unreasonable bulk of the composite addition. The positioning of the composite addition is determined from the survey of the study casts reference to which should be made during the clinical procedure. Specific ultrafine anterior composite materials offer greater flexibility in shade matching and may reduce the potential for abrasion of the clasp arm by the composite though evidence does suggest that this is not a significant problem.

Where doubt exists that the required tooth modification have not been satisfactorarily achieved, an alginate impression can be taken and cast in quick-setting plaster. Surveing this new model will quickly confirm whether or not the preparations are adequate.

All preparation and re-contouring of sound tooth tissue should be completed in enamel. Prepared surfaces should be smoothed, rounded and polished with stones and rubber polishing points of successively reducing coarseness. Although there is little evidence of an increased caries incidence of prepared teeth, many clinicians recommend that fluoride gel or varnish should then be applied to the polished tooth contours. When the final impression is to be made at the same appointment, the application of fluoride should be delayed until the impression has been taken.

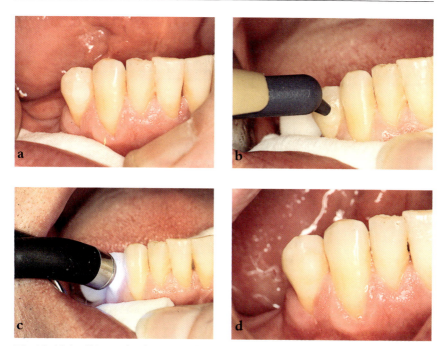

Fig 10-11 (a–d) Use of etch-retained composite to create undercut on the mesiobuccal surface of LR4.

Common errors during tooth preparation

- No or ineffective tooth preparations particularly in relation to the origin of occlusally approaching clasp arms (high survey lines) and where components pass interproximally (embrasure widening).
- Insufficient attention to the occlusion.

Crowning Abutment Teeth

As previously mentioned, crowning of abutment teeth offers the opportunity to create a coronal shape that fulfils all of the requirements of retention and support and provides perfect guiding and reciprocal surfaces (Fig 10-12). Crowning of abutment teeth is indicated when:

- adequate restoration requires coronal coverage

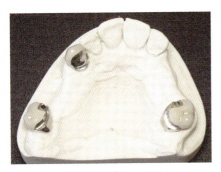

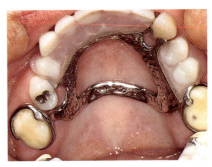

Fig 10-12 Crown abutments incorporating guide surfaces, rests and milled palatal ledges for clasp reciprocal arms on the molar teeth. (Courtesy of Mr D. Barker.)

Fig 10-13 Temporary crowns on UR6 and UL6 fabricated to accommodate an existing partial denture during construction of definitive crowns and a replacement partial denture.

- significant changes to the level of the occlusal plane are planned
- reduction of severe interferences or undercut is required.

Early planning of denture design is essential when multiple crowns or the combined use of fixed and removable prosthesis is intended. Study casts should be surveyed and the denture design established before crown preparation is undertaken. It is only through an awareness of the design of the planned denture and, in particular, its path of insertion that relevant design features can be successfully and predictably incorporated within the crown.

The loads applied by the partial denture – in particular, the clasps – to the crowned abutment tooth necessitate improvements in the retentive and resistance form of the crown preparation. This is achieved by the inclusion of boxes, grooves and pins, and with crown lengthening procedures. Retention and resistance form may be further compromised by the need for additional tooth reduction to accommodate rest seats, guiding surfaces and palatal shoulders for reciprocal clasp arms within the usual coronal form. In general, post-retained crowns do not offer sufficient retention when used to restore clasped abutment teeth and are commonly subject to early failure.

It is usual to construct and fit crowns for abutment teeth before proceeding to the working impression for the partial denture. Transfer of the planned path of insertion from study cast to the die cast on which the crown is constructed is achieved using the transfer tripod points established during the surveying procedure. This requires a full arch impression of the crown(s)

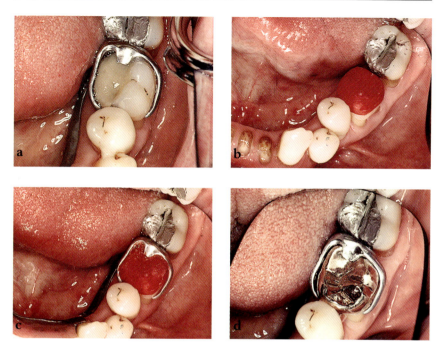

Fig 10-14 (a) LL6 requires restoration with a full veneer gold crown to fit an existing and functioning lower partial denture. (b) Transfer coping on the prepared tooth. (c) The partial denture has been seated and the coping built-up to record the detail of the fitting surface of related components. (d) The completed crown and partial denture.

preparation. In addition, the loss of teeth frequently requires an additional registration stage with wax occlusal rims for a stable jaw relationship record used to articulate working casts prior to crown construction. The continued use of an existing partial denture during fabrication of crowns places particular requirements on the temporisation of prepared teeth. Clearly these must be designed to fit the existing denture but must also resist dislodgement during the normal use and removal of the denture (Fig 10-13).

Construction of crowns to fit an existing partial denture

Crowning of an abutment tooth may be required in the presence of an existing partial denture. A number of techniques to construct the crown so that it fits associated components of the denture have been described. The recommended method involves the use of a transfer coping that is modified intraorally to adapt to the fitting surface of the partial denture (Fig 10-14).

Any necessary clasp undercut is incorporated during the final waxing of the crown in the laboratory.

Key Points

- Commonly required tooth modifications for partial dentures include the preparation of guide surfaces and rest seats, lowering survey lines and the creation of retentive undercut for clasps.
- Tooth preparations are most frequently carried out by simple tooth reshaping. The routine crowning of abutment teeth to achieve an ideal crown shape is not advised.
- Crowning of abutment tooth may be necessary if the tooth is heavily restored or worn. This will provide an ideal opportunity to incorporate any necessary rest seats, retentive undercut or guide surfaces within the crown. This may be predictably achieved only if the path of insertion and final denture design are established before crown preparation is undertaken.

Chapter 11

Clinical Guide IV: Completing and Maintaining the Partial Denture

Aim

This chapter will describe the working impression used for the construction of the metal framework for a partial denture and the clinical stages required to complete the addition of replacement teeth to the framework. It will emphasise the need for scheduled reviews to identify and correct denture errors and to maintain oral health of remaining teeth and denture function.

Outcome

After reading this chapter, the practitioner should be aware of the clinical techniques used for working and altered cast impressions, how to record the definitive jaw relationship and how to try-in and insert the partial denture and the common clinical errors. In addition, the practitioner should be able to recognise the importance of the maintenance of dental health for the long-term function of a partial denture.

Working Impressions

The objectives of this stage are to:
- record a working impression
- complete the laboratory prescription for the construction of the denture framework.

Any preparatory restorative treatment and tooth modifications must be completed before working impressions are recorded. Although rigid, well-extended or modified stock impression trays can be used for the working impression, use of a custom tray constructed on the study cast greatly facilitates the production of a working impression that accurately records the required detail of the remaining teeth and soft tissues and allows the use of a controlled thickness of impression material (Fig 11-1). Modification to the periphery of the custom tray is normally only required when there are gross deficiencies at tray extension or its adaptation over large edentulous areas.

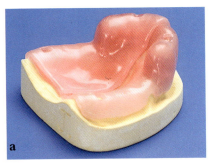
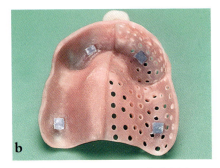

Fig 11-1 Fabrication of custom trays. (a) Wax spacing to ensure a controlled thickness for elastomer and alginate impression materials. (b) The completed custom trays showing a solid and perforated finish for elastomer and alginate impression materials, respectively. Tray stops ensure the accurate and controlled seating of the impression tray.

Such errors normally reflect inadequacies of the preliminary impression. However, when the design of the lower major connector dictates a functional impression of the anterior lingual sulcus, border moulding in this area may be necessary before the working impression is made.

For many cases, and where facilities are immediately available to pour the working cast, alginate will be the impression material of choice. However, its use in the presence of large deep undercut areas frequently results in tearing and distortion of the impression. In such circumstances, and where the cast cannot be poured within 30 minutes, use of a medium-viscosity addition-cured silicone is recommended. More rigid polyether elastomeric impression material should be avoided as the set impression is often difficult to remove from the mouth and will almost certainly result in tooth fracture on removal from the major cast. Regardless of the choice of impression material, large undercut areas that do not need to be recorded should be avoided; this problem can be anticipated by reducing the extension of the custom tray into soft tissue undercut that is not involved in the denture design. A common example is the labial undercut where there are no anterior teeth to be replaced. In this case extension of the tray to just beyond the labial gingival margin is perfectly adequate. Large embrasure spaces should be "filled" with soft carding wax before recording the impression (Fig 11-2).

Common errors
- Impression faults as for preliminary impressions (see Chapter 8), but particularly, overloading the impression of tray.

- Set impression material not firmly adherent to custom tray.
- Incomplete and unclear laboratory design prescription. You get back what you give!

Try-in of the Metal Framework

The objective of this stage is to ensure that the framework fits accurately and does not interfere with the occlusion of the natural teeth.

Before trying the framework in the mouth, check that it fits the master cast and conforms to the prescribed design. Clinically, check the framework's fit, retention and possible occlusal interference, in that order (Fig 11-3).

Minor adjustments are sometimes necessary to ensure the proper seating of the framework. The word minor is stressed. A long period of time spent adjusting a framework is rarely rewarded by a framework that fits satisfacto-

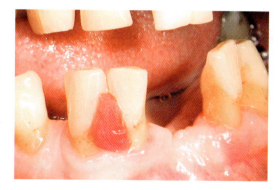

Fig 11-2 Deep embrasure spaces blocked out labially with wax prior to recording the impression.

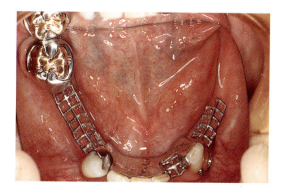

Fig 11-3 Framework try-in.

rily. It is important to adjust only those areas of the framework indicated by the disclosing medium. Do not adjust the finishing edges of plates. Since these are occlusal to the survey line they are unlikely to be the source of error and their adjustment will simply result in a space between the framework and tooth surface. During adjustment, dip the framework in cold water from time to time to avoid overheating and the formation of oxide deposits.

When checking the occlusion, first mark the intercuspal contacts with articulating paper without the framework and then repeat the procedure with the framework seated, but with articulating paper of a different colour. The two sets of contact markings should coincide. When normal intercuspal contacts are reproduced, confirm their presence with shimstock. Repeat the procedure for lateral and protrusive movements. When fitting both upper and lower frameworks, carry out this procedure with one framework, remove it and repeat with the other framework. Finally check the occlusion again with both frameworks in place.

Common errors
- Insufficient attention paid to the occlusion.
- Failure to detect rocking of bounded saddle frameworks. Usually some anteroposterior rocking of a free-end saddle framework with spaced posterior meshwork is possible.

Altered Cast Impression (Lower Free-end Saddle Dentures)

The objective of this clinical stage is to record an impression of the edentulous ridge such that the soft tissues are displaced in the same way as they will be under occlusal loads – the "functional" form of the edentulous ridge. The denture saddle made to this impression will then displace the tissues when seated and no further displacement or movement of the denture base can occur under occlusal loading. This overcomes the problem of differential displacement of the free-end saddle partial denture.

The most common method is to ensure the fit of the denture framework first and then attach a close-fitting temporary free-end saddle base(s) within which the impression of the edentulous ridge is recorded (Fig 11-4). Modification of the temporary base may be required to ensure the correct posterior lingual extension of the saddle acrylic and this is best achieved using green stick compound. Modification is rarely required buccally.

A variety of impression materials can be used to produce equally acceptable results. These include zinc oxide-eugenol impression paste, light-bodied elastomers and impression waxes although the first is perhaps the most convenient. When zinc oxide-eugenol impression paste is used, it is helpful to remove excess impression material from undercuts distal to the abutment teeth before it is set. It is important to rely wholly on the impression material to achieve tissue displacement and seating pressure should only be applied

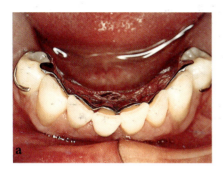

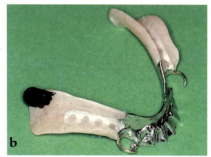

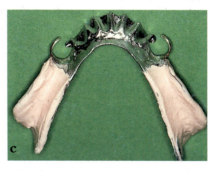

Fig 11-4 The altered cast impression. (a) The framework with close-fitting saddles has been seated and pressure applied over the saddles. The resulting displacement of the saddles has resulted in the connector lifting away from the lingual surfaces of the anterior teeth. If this displacement does not occur and the saddle extensions are acceptable, an altered cast impression is not required. (b) Modification with green stick compound in the posterior lingual area. (c) The completed impression using zinc-oxide/eugenol impression paste.

to that part of the framework supported by the teeth and no pressure should be applied directly to the saddles. This additionally ensures that the framework is fully seated, and remains seated when the impression is made. Excess impression material should be trimmed away from the completed impression and the impression re-seated in the mouth to confirm that the framework was fully seated.

The altered cast impression is used to modify the working cast and the fabrication of the denture is then completed on this modified cast (Fig 11-5).

Besides the theoretical benefit of the altered cast technique, the important practical advantage is that it allows for a more controlled recording of both the denture extension and baring area that is often difficult to achieve with the forms of working impression. It is perhaps this practical rather than the theoretical advantage that results in the improved stability of free-end saddles that is undoubtedly associated with the use of the altered cast technique.

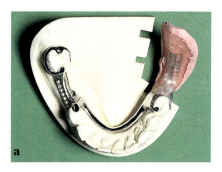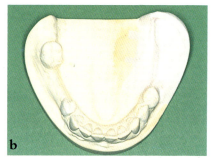

Fig 11-5 (a,b) Modification of the working cast with the altered cast impression.

Common errors
- Buccal overextension and use of too much impression material.
- Framework not fully seated when recording impression.

Definitive Registration

The objectives of this stage are to:
- record the definitive jaw relationships for the partial denture
- select the shade and mould of replacement teeth.

The jaw relationship record should have been previously determined from the examination of the patient and the articulated study casts and the definitive registration simply allows the articulation of the working cast and framework to this relationship (Fig 11-6). As with the preliminary registration, for the vast majority of patients the jaw relationship record will be an existing intercuspal position. If only a few teeth are missing, it may be possible to "hand articulate" accurately the working casts with frameworks without the need for a definitive registration record. More often, addition of wax occlusal rims is necessary to ensure a stable definitive registration. These rims should be trimmed to indicate the required orientation of occlusal planes and buccolingual positions of replacement teeth if this is not clearly indicated by any standing opposing and abutment teeth.

The determination of occlusal face height is required when the partial denture is planned to correct overclosure resulting from tooth wear or the lack of occlusal stops. The new occlusal face height should have been established on the articulated study casts together with tooth-to-tooth relationships at the new height. Reference to the resting face height and freeway space is rarely of practical use when both arches are dentate but is clearly of value when an opposing arch is to be restored with a complete denture.

Selection of tooth mould is frequently not necessary as remaining natural teeth will provide the technician with the necessary information. Shade selection can be problematic and may need to vary with individual replacement teeth to match adjacent standing teeth.

Common errors for this stage are essentially similar to those described for the preliminary registration in Chapter 8.

Partial Denture Try-in

The objective of this stage is to confirm that the arrangement of the replacement teeth restores the correct occlusion and gives a pleasing appearance.

As the majority of partial denture occlusions are designed to conform with and reinforce an existing intercuspal position, the accuracy of the jaw relationships can be established visually and by ensuring normal shimstock contact between opposing natural teeth. Use of articulating paper to confirm

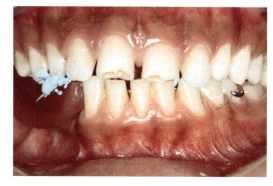

Fig 11-6 A definitive registration recording the intercuspal position as the reference. Normal tooth-to-tooth contacts are present and care has been taken to ensure that denture components such as rests and clasp arms do not interfere with this relationship.

the adequate intercuspation of opposing denture teeth is not normally necessary and carries the risk of displacing denture teeth in the supporting wax of the trial set-up. Minor occlusal errors may be accepted on the assumption that the necessary adjustments can more easily be accomplished when the processed dentures are inserted. Obvious occlusal discrepancies will require a new jaw relation record.

The patient's acceptance of the appearance of the denture in the mouth must be confirmed. Although the correct arrangement, size and colour of the replacement teeth are clearly necessary for a pleasing appearance, the contours of the gingival margins and flanges are as important. In general, the level of the waxed gingival margins should follow that of the natural teeth and the outline of the flanges should follow smooth curves and not end abruptly as straight lines (Fig 11-7).

Any modifications of the set-up prescribed before proceeding directly to processing of the denture should be of a minor nature. Alterations to the set-up following re-registration of jaw relationships or a change of tooth mould and/or shade to improve appearance should be confirmed at a second try-in stage.

Common errors
- Insufficient attention to occlusion.
- The crown length of replacement teeth is too short. This is often seen in the premolar region where a short crown and a low "gingival margin" make denture teeth stand out as artificial, in particular when abutting against a standing canine tooth.

Partial Denture Insert

The objectives of this stage are to:
- check the fit, occlusion and appearance of the completed dentures and to adjust where necessary
- instruct the patient in the correct seating and removal of the dentures
- advise the patient on the proper care of their dentures and to re-emphasise the continued care of the natural teeth.

Before inserting the dentures, check the fitting surface, borders and polished surfaces of the processed acrylic to ensure that there are no projecting nodules or sharp edges and that they have been adequately finished. For examples of good and disappointing completed partial dentures see Fig 11-8. The

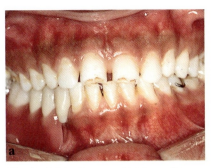
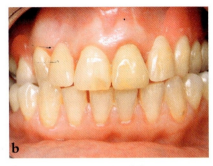

Fig 11-7 Try-in stage. (a) Normal intercuspal contacts are present and the appearance of the replacement teeth is satisfactory. (b) Selection of differing shades for the replacement UR2 and UL2 teeth has resulted in a good match with adjacent teeth. The contour of the left buccal flange blends in well with the soft tissues. The same cannot be said of the replacement UR4 that is too short and looks obviously artificial.

latter is normally the cumulative result of a lack of care and attention to detail throughout the process of denture construction.

Small adjustments of the saddle acrylic (and not the metal framework) may be needed to ensure that the dentures seat fully. Adjust the occlusion as necessary to ensure the correct contact of opposing natural and/or replacement teeth on intercuspation and in lateral and protrusive movements.

The patient should be shown, and have practised, the correct way to take out and insert their dentures. In addition, the patient must be instructed in the use and care of their denture and natural teeth. The need for good plaque control should be emphasised and, where necessary, additional cleaning aids, such as floss, interspace brushes and disclosing tablets should be recommended and their use demonstrated. A review appointment should be made for the following week.

Common errors

- Insufficient attention paid to the occlusion (Fig 11-8c). Normal intercuspal contacts should be verified with shimstock. The denture should remain stable through lateral and protrusive excursive movements which should be smooth and follow the existing tooth guidance where appropriate.
- Denture flange over extension resulting in displacement of the denture in function (Fig 11-8d).

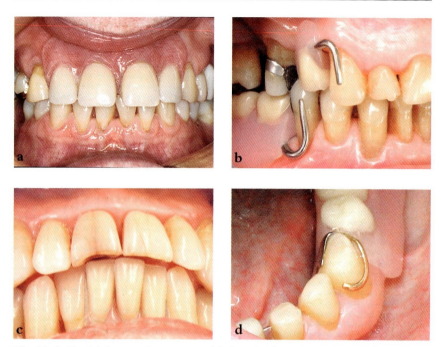

Fig 11-8 Partial denture insert stage. (a) Care in the arrangement of the replacement teeth and the outline and contouring of the labial flange has produced a good aesthetic result. Normal intercuspal contacts have been maintained. (b) Lack of attention to the detail of clasp design, replacement teeth and occlusion has resulted in a disappointing outcome. (c) Normal intercuspal contacts between opposing anterior teeth have not been reproduced. Further occlusal adjustment is necessary. (d) Flange overextension in relation to the buccal fraenum.

Review and Maintenance

The objectives of this stage are to:
- identify and correct any errors of occlusion or of fit which may have caused discomfort
- check and reinforce the patient's oral and denture hygiene
- ensure the continued maintenance of denture function.

At the review, the mouth should be examined for signs of denture-related injury whether or not the patient complains of discomfort. Discomfort commonly results from excessive pressure applied to teeth and the soft tissues from a tight fitting framework or errors in the fit and/or extension of the saddles, respectively. The areas requiring adjustment should be identified with

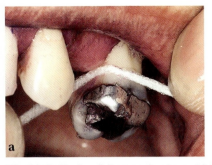 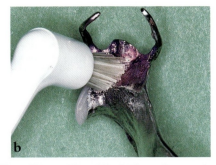

Fig 11-9 Oral and denture hygiene. (a) Use of Super Floss (Oral-B) on the proximal surface of an abutment tooth. (b) A single tufted brush for cleaning intricate areas of the denture framework.

suitable disclosing media. Excessive pressures on both teeth and soft tissues may also result from occlusal errors, and the occlusion should always be checked before the denture is relieved over sore areas. Where adjustments have been necessary, a further review should normally be arranged.

The patient's oral and denture hygiene should be checked and, if necessary, reinforced. Areas of concern are those covered by and abutting the denture and, in particular, abutment teeth. Instruction in the use of additional oral hygiene aids such as Super Foss (Oral-B) and single tufted brushes may be required (Fig 11-9).

The long-term function of a partial denture will be compromised by the deformation and eventual fracture of denture components, by denture tooth fracture and wear and by the continued resorption of the edentulous ridge. Adjustments and repairs to clasps and the repair of fractured denture teeth are commonly required. Deterioration in the fit of a partial denture resulting from continued bone resorption is a particular feature of free-end saddle dentures and is corrected by simple reline procedures when increasing instability is noted. Reline impressions should be recorded with the denture out of occlusion but with firm pressure applied to the framework to ensure its proper seating. Important as this maintenance is to the continued satisfactory function of a partial denture, it should always be remembered that the long-term success of a partial denture will be determined by the success in establishing a healthy oral environment prior to denture construction, and to the maintenance of oral health once the denture has been fitted.

Key Points

Care and attention to detail at all clinical stages in the construction of partial dentures are necessary. In particular, this includes the following:

- Well-designed custom impression trays to facilitate accurate working impressions.
- An altered cast impression to improve the fit and stability of lower free-end denture saddles.
- Attention to the occlusion at all clinical stages.
- Selection of the appropriate shade and size of replacement teeth.
- Care in the shaping and contouring of associated acrylic flanges.

Index

Quintessentials for General Dental Practitioners Series

in 36 volumes

Editor-in-Chief: Professor Nairn H F Wilson

The Quintessentials for General Dental Practitioners Series covers basic principles and key issues in all aspects of modern dental medicine. Each book can be read as a stand-alone volume or in conjunction with other books in the series.

Publication date,
approximately

Oral Surgery and Oral Medicine, Editor: John G Meechan

Practical Dental Local Anaesthesia	available
Practical Oral Medicine	Autumn 2004
Practical Conscious Sedation	available
Practical Surgical Dentistry	Autumn 2004

Imaging, Editor: Keith Horner

Interpreting Dental Radiographs	available
Panoramic Radiology	Autumn 2004
Twenty-first Century Dental Imaging	Autumn 2004

Periodontology, Editor: Iain L C Chapple

Understanding Periodontal Diseases: Assessment and Diagnostic Procedures in Practice	available
Decision-Making for the Periodontal Team	available
Successful Periodontal Therapy – A Non-Surgical Approach	available
Periodontal Management of Children, Adolescents and Young Adults	available
Periodontal Medicine: A Window on the Body	Autumn 2005

Implantology, Editor: Lloyd J Searson

Implantology in General Dental Practice	Autumn 2004
Managing Orofacial Pain in Practice	Summer 2005

Endodontics, Editor: John M Whitworth

Rational Root Canal Treatment in Practice	available
Managing Endodontic Failure in Practice	available
Managing Dental Trauma in Practice	Autumn 2004
Preventing Pulpal Injury in Practice	Summer 2005

Prosthodontics, Editor: P Finbarr Allen

Teeth for Life for Older Adults	available
Complete Dentures – from Planning to Problem Solving	available
Removable Partial Dentures	available
Fixed Prosthodontics in Dental Practice	Autumn 2004
Occlusion: A Theoretical and Team Approach	Summer 2005

Operative Dentistry, Editor: Paul A Brunton

Decision-Making in Operative Dentistry	available
Aesthetic Dentistry	available
Indirect Restorations	Autumn 2004
Psychological and Behavioural Management of Adult Dental Patients	Autumn 2004
Applied Dental Materials in Operative Dentistry	Spring 2005

Paediatric Dentistry/Orthodontics, Editor: Marie Therese Hosey

Child Taming: How to Cope with Children in Dental Practice	available
Paediatric Cariology	Autumn 2004
Treatment Planning for the Developing Dentition	Autumn 2004

General Dentistry and Practice Management, Editor: Raj Rattan

The Business of Dentistry	available
Risk Management	available
Practice Management for the Dental Team	Autumn 2004
Quality Assurance	Autumn 2004
Dental Practice Design	Summer 2005
IT in Dentistry: A Working Manual	Autumn 2005

Quintessence Publishing Co. Ltd., London